Health and Illness in the Community

Oxford Core Texts

Health and Illness in the Community

an Oxford Core Text

Edited by
Ross J Taylor
Blair H Smith
Edwin R van Teijlingen

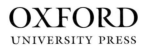

OXFORD
UNIVERSITY PRESS

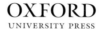

OXFORD
UNIVERSITY PRESS

Great Clarendon Street, Oxford OX2 6DP

Oxford University Press is a department of the University of Oxford.
It furthers the University's objective of excellence in research, scholarship,
and education by publishing worldwide in

Oxford New York

Auckland Bangkok Buenos Aires Cape Town, Chennai
Dar es Salaam Delhi Hong Kong Istanbul Karachi Kolkata
Kuala Lumpur Madrid Melbourne Mexico City Mumbai Nairobi
São Paulo Shanghai Taipei Tokyo Toronto

Oxford is a registered trade mark of Oxford University Press
in the UK and in certain other countries

Published in the United States
by Oxford University Press Inc., New York

A catalogue record for this title is available from the British Library

Library of Congress Cataloguing in Publication Data
Data available
ISBN 0-19-263168-3

10 9 8 7 6 5 4 3 2 1

Typeset by Newgen Imaging Systems (P) Ltd., Chennai, India
Printed in Italy
on acid-free paper by
Legoprint

Foreword

This book is about the context within which illness is experienced, health is sought, and medicine is practised. It shows us that the determinants of health and illness are much wider than the influence of medicine or, indeed, health-care. Practitioners rightly focus attention on the individual seeking care during an episode of illness. However, it is generally recognized that the effectiveness of clinical decisions made for each patient is increased if the doctor takes account of the patient's family and community setting. Equally, the impact of these decisions is mediated through the environmental, economic, and political conditions of the day.

Medical education has undergone a radical overhaul in the last decade following the publication of *Tomorrow's Doctors* by the General Medical Council. The importance of the community and the health of the population has been emphasized, and there are moves to include the assessment of these aspects of medicine into summative assessments. At the same time the impact of medical schools on local and national life, and their social accountability, has been widely debated. As a result the undergraduate curriculum has become more relevant to the identification of the common and important diseases seen in the UK today, while addressing the complexity of managing disease and illness in our diverse modern society. This has been underpinned by an explicit definition of the qualities required for all UK registered doctors in the GMC publication *Good Medical Practice*, which includes a recognition of the tension between providing care for individuals, and seeking to improve the overall health and well-being of populations.

In this book the reader is introduced to the structures and processes in society that influence healthcare. The practitioner can identify ways in which their own decisions can be enhanced and improved, whilst on a practical level some of the surprising outcomes from encounters and interventions may become clearer. Medical students can begin to appreciate the breadth of medical practice, and reach a deeper understanding of both its power and its limitations.

Dame Lesley Southgate

Professor of General Practice and Medical Education
Royal Free and University College Medical School (RFUCMS)
President of Royal College of General Practitioners

Acknowledgements

We are grateful to everybody who has been involved in the Community Course at the University of Aberdeen Medical School for feedback, comments, observations, and criticisms on that course. We are particularly grateful to the students, tutors, and external examiners: their involvement has helped shape this textbook.

We are also grateful to George Deans and Monika Watt, who contributed significantly to the editorial process of this book during their time in the Department of General Practice & Primary Care, and the Department of Environmental and Occupational Medicine, University of Aberdeen, respectively. Finally, we are grateful to Netta Clark, who typed the manuscript and provided general assistance with the collection of material.

Copyright permission

Contents

Contributors

Clifford Eastmond
Consultant Physician
Aberdeen Royal Infirmary
Foresterhill
Aberdeen
AB25 220

Philip Hannaford
Grampian Health Board
Professor of Primary Care
University of Aberdeen
Foresterhill Health Centre
Westburn Road
Aberdeen
AB25 2AY

Peter Helms
Professor of Child Health
University of Aberdeen
Foresterhill
Aberdeen
AB25 2ZD

Mhoira Leng
Consultant in Palliative Care
Roxburghe House
North Deeside Road
Aberdeen
AB13 0HR

Linda McKie
Research Professor in Sociology
Glasgow Caledonian University
Cowcaddens Road
Glasgow
G4 0BA

Gwyn D. Seymour
Professor of Medicine (Care of the
Elderly)

University of Aberdeen
Foresterhill Health Centre
Westburn Road
Aberdeen
AB25 2AY

Ruth Seymour
Consultant in Rehabilitation
Medicine
Woodend Hospital
Eday Road
Aberdeen
AB15 2XF

Blair H. Smith
Senior Lecturer in General Practice
University of Aberdeen
Foresterhill Health Centre
Westburn Road
Aberdeen
AB25 2AY

W. Cairns Smith
Professor of Public Health
University of Aberdeen
Foresterhill
Aberdeen
AB25 2ZD

Ross J. Taylor
Senior Lecturer in General Practice
University of Aberdeen
Foresterhill Health Centre
Westburn Road
Aberdeen
AB25 2AY

Edwin R. van Teijlingen
Senior Lecturer in Public Health
University of Aberdeen

Medical School
Foresterhill
Aberdeen
AB25 2ZD

Lawrence Whalley
Professor of Mental Health
University of Aberdeen
Foresterhill
Aberdeen
AB25 2ZD

Fiona L. R. Williams
Senior Lecturer
University of Dundee
Ninewells Hospital and Medical
School
Dundee
DD1 9SY

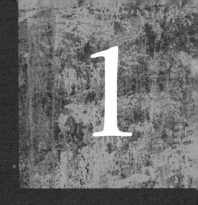

1

CHAPTER 1

Introduction: society, health, and illness

CHAPTER 1

Introduction: society, health, and illness

CASE 1

Phil is a medical student attached to the children's ward of the teaching hospital, where he has just finished his study of a 7-year-old patient, Jane. He established that Jane was admitted 2 days previously with a bad asthma attack. On admission she had been very breathless and distressed, but now, after treatment and observation, her lung function is back to normal, her breathing is easy, and she is much happier. Phil tells the consultant tutor that Jane has made a full recovery and should now go home and because she is so well there is no need to arrange a follow-up appointment for Jane.

Phil has not established the full facts. Jane's mother abuses alcohol and is drunk most days from around 3pm. Jane's respiratory distress had been discovered by a neighbour who had found her mother unconscious at the same time. The house was filthy, with overflowing bins and ashtrays, empty vodka bottles, and no food. Jane's father, who had abandoned the family 2 years ago, had been contacted on her admission, and has been spending many hours with her. He is talking of re-establishing a paternal relationship.

The consultant, although pleased with Phil's summary of Jane's physical condition, decides that it is too early to discharge Jane. He decides to contact other professionals with a view to Jane's long-term health and keeps her in the ward meantime.

Medicine happens in hospitals and health centres. People go there from the community, become patients, then, if they are lucky, go home again cured or patched up.

Figure 1.1 represents the traditional view, held by most members of the public and by many doctors, and therefore the one brought to medical school by most prospective members of the profession. In this book, we argue that this is only one small, though very important, part of medicine. A broader appreciation of the nature of the profession and its practice requires study of health and illness as it occurs, and is experienced in the community. However, hospitals and health centres are but a part of this community and hospital care should not necessarily be seen as outside community care. Hospitals are

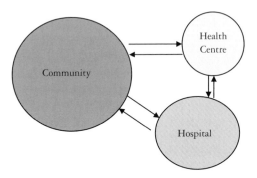

Fig. 1.1 Traditional view of the link between hospital, health centre and community.

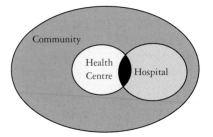

Fig. 1.2 Alternative view of the link between hospital, health centre and community.

part of the overall health service provision and represent one of several facilities in the community that a person might use in order to manage life with a chronic medical condition (see Fig. 1.2). In this view, hospitals and health centres are seen as closely related and interacting parts of an over-all community.

A background understanding of where a person comes from, his or her family, housing, lifestyle, culture, and internal motivation will allow a doctor to appreciate, for example, the importance of the illness she is treating and the significance of the treatment to the patient. Without such an understanding, he/she can only treat an illness, not a person. This understanding is important for *all* doctors, not just general practitioners or community health specialists.

Medical students, therefore, must have a solid education in behavioural science (e.g. psychology and sociology), as well as in bio-medical science (e.g. anatomy and physiology). In other words, it is important for us to understand how an individual functions internally (psychologically and physiologically) *and* externally, in relation to other human beings. It is also important not to see people in isolation, since groups of these human beings form families, communities, and societies. Such cultural institutions have a major impact on the actions and reactions of individuals.

In Case 1 it is clear that to have treated Jane's asthma successfully in clinical terms was only to have treated her superficially. A full knowledge of the case (i.e. the person) reveals that there is much, much more still to do, but provides clues to a way forward. Deployment of health professionals based in the community, such as Jane's general practitioner, the health visitor, the social work department, and the community mental health team, all in liaison with the hospital consultant, can lead towards an optimistic outcome for Jane and her family. Had she been discharged, as Phil suggested, the outlook would have been bleak. Jane's family circumstances are important in understanding how Jane got in the condition she is in now and how best to improve her health. However, there are also wider issues at play related to the community of which Jane is a part.

Perhaps the major purpose of this book is to help you to develop empathy; that is, the ability to understand the position of another person. If this book helps you, now or in the future, to understand more deeply the position of patients or clients that you will come to deal with as a healthcare worker, it will have achieved that end.

Medicine in the community

Having argued that hospital care is part of the wider community of care, we have to ask ourselves: 'What exactly do we mean by community?' Everybody will have an intuitive perception of what constitutes a community, and everybody's definition will be slightly, if not considerably, different. In *The Concise Oxford Dictionary of Current English*, one of the definitions for 'community' is:

> organized political, municipal, or social body; body of people living in same locality, etc., in common, (*the immigrant mercantile, Jewish community*). The public; monastic, socialist, etc., body practising community of goods; body of nations unified by common interests . . .

However, dictionary definitions are not always all that helpful when it comes to terms as vague as 'community', 'society', or 'democracy'. There are different ways of defining a community, the four most commonly defining factors are:

◆ locality;
◆ culture;
◆ social stratification;
◆ functional groups.

Locality

A community might be defined on a geographical or neighbourhood basis. Community policing fits under this definition, so does a neighbourhood watch scheme, or the Morningside community in Edinburgh or a community pharmacy. The underlying assumption is that people living in the same area have similar concerns, owing to their geographical proximity. Jane is part of a community in a neighbourhood, since it was a neighbour who found her.

Culture

Communities may be defined in cultural terms, such as the 'Chinese' or 'Asian' community in Britain, the 'Irish' community in London, or the 'Dutch' community in Aberdeen. Here, the assumption is that common cultural traditions are more important than locality boundaries or other barriers, and unite otherwise scattered and disparate groups of people. There is an expectation that members of a cultural group will help each other and share resources, or at least share information about such resources. Jane's ethnic background is not given, but it is easy to see that Jane could be part of such a community.

Social stratification

A community may be based on structural interests held in common, which are usually the product of social stratification. Thus, we have 'the working class community' or 'women'. Community is based on notions of power, status, and ascribed roles in society. This definition implies that members of a community share networks of support, knowledge, and resources, which may transcend other boundaries, even national ones. Jane is part of a lone-parent family, the number of which is increasing mainly as a result of changes in British society, since far more couples divorce than ever before. Moreover, women head nine out of 10 one-parent families, and well over half of these women and their children are living in poverty (Millar 1987).

Functional groups

A community may be based on functional interests held in common, which are usually the product of one particular common interest. Thus, we have the 'gay community' or 'Jehovah's witnesses'. As with the previous definition, this definition also implies that members of a community share networks of support, knowledge, and resources that may transcend other boundaries, even national ones. Jane's mother might be thinking about joining Alcoholic Anonymous (AA), an international functional group.

It is immediately obvious that individuals will often belong to more than one community. Black working class women are likely to live in certain neighbourhoods (location), they belong to an ethnic group (culture), and they are part of the working class, as well as women (both social stratification). White pensioners in Birmingham's suburbia also belong to different communities, some of which may or may not overlap with the black working class women. Being part of a community is not something that is static. In reality we see that people move between different communities during their lifetime. People move physically from one area to another, but they might also move from one social group to another, or from one functional group to another (e.g. from students to doctors or from being members of a students' union to being a member of a trade union) and people might be socially mobile within the social stratification. Thus, a student from a working class family in a rural area in the Scottish Highlands might move to become a middle-class doctor in suburban Newcastle.

> The main point to bear in mind is that 'community' could mean something different to different people and that people could be part of several different communities at the same time.

Medical education in Britain takes place in medical schools, nearly all of which are linked to academic hospitals. It makes sense in terms of efficiency to concentrate teaching in a place where there are many patients (i.e. teaching material). However, concentrating the teaching in hospitals also distorts our view of what students and doctors do in Medicine. The case study at the beginning of this chapter indicates that it is very easy for a medical student to focus on the patient as presented in hospital, without considering the wider social and cultural background of that patient.

In this book we examine health and illness in the context of the community. We begin with an examination of the 'nature' of health, of illness, and of society (Part 1). Then we examine some of the factors that influence health in society (Part 2). We conclude by examining the impact of health in society and the ways in which society adapts to this (Part 3).

Part 1 sets the content for the practice of medicine in the community. It begins with a description of the society in which we live, including its constituents and the implications of these. Then the diseases and illnesses that affect our society will be described, in order to explain the challenge that we face in the medical profession. We precede a discussion of what we actually mean by illness and why people consult doctors, with the essential first step of attempting to define health.

SUMMARY POINTS

- Traditionally, most medical education has taken place in hospitals where there are many patients (teaching material), mostly with more serious illnesses.
- Hospitals deal with only certain kinds and stages of illness so that traditional medical education provides a greatly distorted picture of illness as a whole.
- People live in communities, which may be defined in many different ways, and their illnesses need to be viewed in the context of their way of life.
- Community care should not be seen as opposite to hospital care. Ideally, they are both an integrated part of overall provision of health services.
- The balance of provision of health care in hospital or in community care is, therefore, not fixed, but subject to constant change.

References and further reading

Last, J. (2001). *A Dictionary of Epidemiology*, 4th edn. Oxford University Press, Oxford.

Millar, J. (1987). 'Lone mothers'. In: *Women and Poverty in Britain* (eds C. Glendinning & J. Millar). Wheatsheaf Books Ltd, Brighton.

Sykes, J.B. (1986). *The Concise Oxford Dictionary of Current English*, 7th edn. Oxford University Press, Oxford.

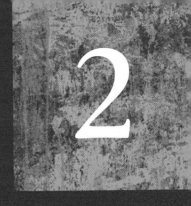

2

CHAPTER 2
Description of society

CHAPTER 2
Description of society

Introduction

You might wonder why we bother describing our society, because with the notable exception of the relatively small number of doctors working in Public Health, Occupational Medicine, and Environmental Health, doctors generally deal with individual patients, who receive personal care. As outlined in the previous chapter it is important to recognize that each person is not an isolated individual, but forms part of a wider group, be it a family, a local community, or a nation. Anything that affects an individual is likely to have an influence on such larger groups. Equally, events or forces that affect societies and communities are likely to have an effect on individuals in those groups. It is necessary to consider the environment in which the individual lives and works in order to have a better understanding of their health and their health-related behaviour.

CASE 1

A 'problem family' is removed by the local council from a housing estate. As a result of this action the remaining residents feel far less stressed, one neighbour of the 'problem family' now no longer needs her sleeping tablets, and the 7-year-old daughter of an upstairs neighbour stops wetting her bed.

In this case (1) without physical changes or medical intervention, the quality of life of a number of local residents improves due to changes in their social environment.

Organization of society

The way a society organizes its political system has an influence on people's lives and their health. Political decisions will have an impact on the organization and funding of health care, but will also have an impact on wider issues, which in themselves might influence people's health. If health care is largely state-funded, as it is in Britain, the Secretary of State for Health needs to battle with other ministers in the Cabinet for resources, playing off health care provision against, for example, education and defence. Thus, a Cabinet decision to provide more money to train more customs officers could mean that less money is made available to reduce the waiting list for people with hip operations.

Health care systems all over the world seem to be facing a funding crisis. This is not simply a question of allocation of scarce resources, but also of political decision-making and priorities. For example, political decisions regarding road safety, such as introducing a maximum speed on the motorway or making it compulsory to wear a seat belt in a car, have an impact on the number of serious accidents on our roads. More indirectly, they have an impact on the availability of kidneys for transplants, because these road safety measures lead to fewer deaths on the road.

On a larger scale, the political decision to provide national health services through the NHS (National Health Service) in Britain (see also Chapter 14) has an influence on our health. In a tax-funded health care system such as the NHS there are few incentives for doctors to do 'unnecessary' operations/interventions to be able to charge their patient more, because patients do not directly pay the doctor, and the doctor is not reimbursed by the number of operations or procedures conducted.

Work

The average person in an industrialized society spends a considerable amount of time working. Work in everyday language is often taken to mean paid employment, but we could include unpaid employment such as work carried out at home by homemakers ('housewives'), students, prisoners, etc. In Britain, approximately 74% of the population aged 16–64 is in paid employment (or seeking paid employment). The remaining quarter of the adult population comprises retired people, students, and homemakers. Men are still more likely to be economically active than women, although the proportion of men who are economically active has dropped from about 90 to 85% between 1971 and 1998, whilst the proportion of women has increased from about 55% to over 70% in the same period.

Paid employment provides people with an income, but work also offers people non-financial benefits, such as social contacts, status, and a purpose in life. For example, being a doctor is not simply a job that pays a salary—it provides a certain status in society. It also provides social contacts, some very close contacts if you consider the number of doctors who are in relationships with colleagues, such as other doctors, nurses, midwives, etc. Work also provides a purpose in life. When we meet new people we often ask, after we have found out their names, 'And what do you do?' The importance of work as a provider of purpose in life is often not recognized until it is no longer there. When people lose their job and become unemployed or retire, sometimes a sense of 'what am I going to do?' occurs. Thus, we often observe an increase in mental health problems in people who become unemployed, especially if the period of unemployment is lengthy.

Not all work is the same

We use people's work, especially paid employment, as an indicator for social class. One way of describing our society is using socio-economic classes (see Chapter 7). Socio-economic classes are based on people's occupation. Similar occupations are grouped together: thus, professional occupations such as lawyers, doctors, and company directors are grouped together in one social class, whilst manual occupations such as road sweepers, gardeners, and hospital porters are grouped together in another social class. The main social class/occupational classification currently used in the UK is listed in Chapter 7. What is important for people with an interest in health is that different occupational groups appear to have different life chances. For example, people in 'manual' socio-economic groups face higher risks of unemployment, coronary heart attacks, imprisonment, poverty, or giving birth to a low-birth weight baby. This social inequality in health is attracting increasing fundamental attention and is discussed further in Part 2.

Different jobs have different effects on people's health. Such effects can be short-term, as well as long-term and direct, as well as indirect (Table 2.1). Some short-term effects are clearly attributable to the work/workplace of an individual, for example, physical accidents at work, whilst others are more difficult to attribute, for example, excessive alcohol consumption at business lunches, which leads to problem drinking and alcoholism. One could argue that, for example, a particular doctor might not have ended up with a drinking problem if he/she had opted for a career in teaching. The longer-term direct effects of work on an individual may sometimes be more difficult to trace back to work. Stress-related illness might be difficult to link to someone's occupation, because the person might have a personality that is susceptible to stress or experience stress at home due to relationship problem. Thus, it is difficult to relate mental health problems to years of stress at work (see Chapter 16 for a further discussion of this). On the other hand, pneumoconiosis in underground coal miners and industrial deafness in certain groups of factory workers are very clear examples of occupational diseases.

Table 2.1 The nature of occupational diseases

	Directly attributable	Indirectly attributable
Short-term	Accident at work	An episode of problem drinking
Long-term	Industrial deafness	Coronary heart disease due to stress at work

Environment

The environment can be defined in different ways. There is the natural geological environment in which we live—the land, the sea, the rivers—but also the geographical environment, the cities, the countryside, the motorway system. The environment can also be seen as our human/social environment: the people who live in our street and the fellow students on our course. Finally, the environment can be seen as something more philosophical and idealistic, e.g. the flora and fauna on this planet that have to be saved and protected from human interventions. Here, and especially in Chapter 9 'Environmental influences on health', we consider the first two types of definition.

Culture and structure of society

Our multi-ethnic culture is constantly changing. For example, nuclear families are in decline: more people are living alone, there are more single parent families, most lone-parent families are headed by a woman, and so on.

Our work and leisure patterns are also changing. Many people in Britain have more time and money available for leisure. We work on average fewer hours per week than our grandparents. We have more spare time. In our spare time we watch more television than our parents and have a more sedentary lifestyle. We have more holidays and travel further afield. Consequently, we have more experience of other cultures, universal events, and universal culture. Our children will have seen more deaths on television by the time they are 15 than our grandparents will have seen in a lifetime.

The media and health

The media, especially newspapers, television, radio, movies, and the Internet, help shape people's views and attitudes. Television programmes, such as the American soap opera ER (which stands for 'emergency room'), provide people with an experience and, subsequently, with certain expectations about their health and health care. According to the Scottish Ambulance Services, who are the main training agency in cardiac resuscitation in Scotland, more people have attempted such resuscitation than there are trained in it. The likely explanation is that people are picking up the technique from television programmes and films portraying resuscitation. One of the risks is, of course, that people 'think' they know what to do, but in fact do not resuscitate correctly.

Transport and health

Another major change in our society over the past century has been the increase in motorized transport. It is hard to believe that the automobile is barely 100 years old and the aeroplane even less than that. People travel more and further than ever before. Every year there are more cars on the road in the UK. Today, unlike in the recent past, more children are driven to school than walk or cycle. Although there are more cars on the road, the proportion of those that are involved in fatal traffic accidents is going down. Our roads are safer, our cars are getting safer, perhaps drivers are getting more experienced too.

Recreational drug use: an example of lifestyle

Drugs are widely used in our society. Most people use caffeine (coffee, tea, cola, and 'energy' drinks) on a daily basis. Many adults and teenagers use alcohol and a smaller proportion use tobacco. These drugs are, of course, legal in our society and alcohol is very much part of everyday life. One indication as to how integrated and 'normal' alcohol use is was highlighted in a systematic study of the contents of 50 television programmes shown on British television. This study in the late 1980s found that four out of five programmes contained visual or verbal references to alcohol. On average, there was a reference to alcohol every 6 min. The television programmes showed more alcohol being consumed than soft drinks, but there were few references to the hazards of alcohol consumption (Smith *et al*. 1988).

A recent content analysis of the portrayal of smoking in 50 Hollywood films starring 10 popular actresses revealed that leading actresses were as likely to smoke in movies aimed at young people as at adult audiences. However, films certified as suitable for young people were *less* likely than adult-rated movies to contain negative message about smoking (Escamilla *et al*. 2000).

Estimates of illegal drug use suggest that cannabis (or marijuana) is the most widely misused recreational drug in Britain. It is estimated that over 40% of 15- and 16-year-olds have, at some time, used illicit drugs (mainly cannabis). Other drugs used illegally include opium derivatives [morphine, heroin, methadone, diconal, and DF118 (dihydrocodeine)], benzodiazepines (diazepam and temazepam), and ecstasy.

If we consider changes over time in drug use we see that smoking is becoming less acceptable in many industrialized societies, with the introduction of bans on smoking in public places and legislation against tobacco advertising on television. However, at the same time we see that the portrayal of tobacco in films is still very acceptable and is more positive in films aimed at younger people, who are more vulnerable in terms of likelihood of taking up smoking. At the same time we see a relaxation of attitudes towards the use of so-called soft drugs in many countries. Irrespective of whether recreational drugs are legal or illegal, they are likely to have an impact on people's health and, subsequently, on the utilization of health services.

SUMMARY POINTS

◆ Society is gradually, but constantly changing.

◆ The acts of individuals may affect society and vice versa. Everyone forms part of a series of groups—the family, the local community, the nation.

◆ The way a society organizes its political system can have an influence on people's lives and their health, e.g. through how it funds health services, its attitude to work and to unemployment, to protection of the environment, and to enhancement of life-style and culture.

◆ The media helps to shape society.

◆ The chapter gives a number of specific examples, illustrating also how societies are constantly evolving and, to an extent, becoming more universal in their outlook.

References and further reading

Porter, M., Alder, B., & Abraham, C. (eds) (1999). *Psychology and Sociology Applied to Medicine: an illustrated colour text*. Churchill Livingstone, Edinburgh.

Escamilla, G., Cradock, A.L., & Kawachi, I. (2000). Women and smoking in Hollywood movies: a content analysis, *American Journal of Public Health*, 90, 412–414.

Moon, G. & Gillespie, R. (eds) (1995). *Society and Health: an introduction to social science for health professionals*. Routledge, London.

Smith, C., Roberts, J.L., Pendelton, L.L. (1988). The portrayal of alcohol on British television: a content analysis. *Health Education Research*, 3, 267–272.

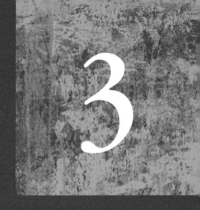

3

CHAPTER 3

An epidemiological picture of society

An epidemiological picture of society

In the previous chapter, we described a profile of the society in which we live. In this chapter, we will explore the nature and types of illness occurring in this society, using the numerical science of epidemiology. Epidemiology is 'the study of the distribution and determinants of health-related states or events in specified populations, and the application of this study to control health problems' (Last, 2001).

Crucially, this study must take account of the specific time, place, and person affected as the distribution and determinants will vary greatly with these. For example, the rate of occurrence of heart disease is very different between eighteenth century English women and twentieth century Finnish men. Understanding these differences has helped with design of prevention and treatment.

Looking for differences

In essence, epidemiology involves comparing groups (often called study populations) in order to detect differences that provide:

♦ pointers as to what might be causing illness (aetiological clues);

♦ the scope for prevention;

♦ the identification of high risk or priority groups within society who may benefit from an intervention.

The study populations may be defined by place of residence, age, gender, ethnic origin, lifestyle, workplace, use of a particular healthcare service, or some other characteristic. Sometimes the same groups are compared at different points in time. The comparisons frequently involve calculating how often an event occurs in each group so that differences between groups are revealed. In other types of study, the characteristics of different groups are measured and compared in order to see whether there is an important association between a characteristic and a disease. Risk factors are those characteristics found to be associated with a particular disease.

Nearly 50 years ago, the first strong evidence of the harmful effects of smoking was beginning to emerge. Several studies compared the smoking habits of individuals with lung cancer with those of people without; a major association between cigarette smoking and lung cancer was found. However, showing that an association exists is not the same as saying that the risk factor caused the disease. There may be many other explanations for an association, although in the case of smoking few would now dispute that smoking causes lung cancer and many other diseases. Epidemiological data need to be interpreted carefully, especially when used to inform clinical and public health decisions.

Measures of disease occurrence

Box 1 contains definitions for some common event rates. It is important that these terms are used consistently so that everyone is clear about what exactly is being compared. When calculating event rates, only people at risk of developing the disease (i.e. the population at risk) should be included. Thus, a study of cancer of the testes should not include females in the population at risk.

BOX 1 Some common event rates

Incidence

The number of new events (e.g. new cases of illness) occurring in a defined population within a specified period of time. It is usually expressed as a rate, such as the annual breast cancer rate in the United Kingdom (UK) per 100,000 women. This incidence rate would be calculated by:

(Number of new cases of breast cancer registered in the UK in a given year $\times 100,000$)/(Number of women living in the UK during the year)

More generally, incidence rates are calculated by:

(Number of new events in a specified period $\times 10^n$)/(Number of persons at risk during this period)

Prevalence

The total number of events in a defined population at a designated time. It is important to specify the time period. Point prevalence describes the situation at a particular point in time (for example, at the time that a health survey was conducted). Annual prevalence describes the total number of events at any time during one year. It includes old cases arising before, but extending into the year under consideration, as well as new cases occurring during the same year. Events arising before, but not extending into the year, because they resolve or result in death, are not included. Lifetime prevalence describes the total number of persons known to have an event for at least part of their life.

Prevalence is usually expressed as a prevalence rate, calculated by:

(Number of all events in specified period $\times 10^n$)/(Number of persons at risk during this period)

BOX 1 Continued

Morbidity rate

The incidence of non-fatal cases of disease in a given population in a specified period.

Mortality rate

The incidence of fatal cases of disease in a given population in a specified period. Often all-cause mortality is broken down into cause-specific mortality rates, although this does make important assumptions about how well clinicians can accurately determine, and document, what someone dies from. A cause-specific mortality rate would be calculated by:

(Number of deaths attributed to that cause in specified period $\times$ 10^n)/(Number of persons at risk of dying during this period)

Crude rate

This is the incidence, prevalence or mortality rate calculated by the simple formulae given above.

Adjusted rate

Comparing crude rates can be misleading if the groups being compared are very different from each other. Event rates, therefore, are often adjusted so that they reflect the rates that would have occurred if each group had a common (standard) structure. For example, age-standardized cancer rates are rates of cancer that would occur if the population had a standard age structure.

Incidence and prevalence rates are closely related. Prevalence rates depend on how many people:

- develop the disease (i.e. the incidence rates);
- die from the disease;
- recover from the disease.

(see Fig. 3.1)

Many diseases (such as the common cold) occur frequently, but are usually short-lived with complete recovery; their incidence rates tend to be high, but their prevalence rates low. Other diseases (such as diabetes) occur less frequently, but once present are permanent; their incidence rates tend to be low, but their prevalence rates high.

Prevalence rates are affected by a number of factors unrelated to the cause of disease, such as those influencing recovery or survival after the onset of the disease. Ideally, studies trying to understand the cause of disease should use incident, rather than prevalent cases of disease. Prevalence rates are more useful for assessing the need for health care services in a population and for the planning of medical services.

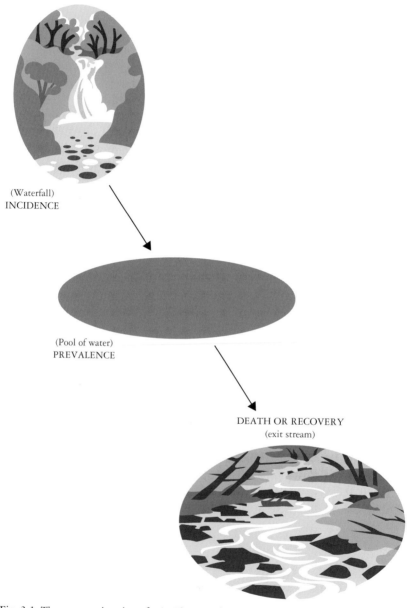

(Waterfall)
INCIDENCE

(Pool of water)
PREVALENCE

DEATH OR RECOVERY
(exit stream)

Fig. 3.1 The waterpool analogy for incidence and prevalence of disease.

Geographical comparisons

Many studies compare the rate of disease in different geographical locations (e.g. different cities, regions, or countries). Figure 3.2 shows estimated age-adjusted incidence and mortality rates for breast cancer in 15 European

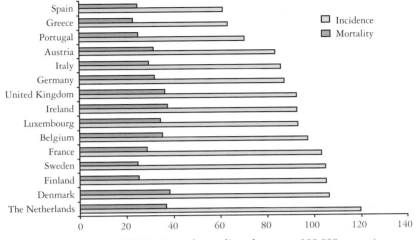

Fig. 3.2 Breast cancer in 1995 (estimated age-adjusted rates per 100,000 women).

countries. Although breast cancer is the most common cancer to affect women in all of the countries shown, the figure shows considerable variations in disease occurrence between the countries. Thus, in 1995 the incidence of breast cancer among women living in the Netherlands was almost twice that observed in women from Spain. In other words, women living in the Netherlands apparently had nearly twice the risk of developing breast cancer compared with women living in Spain. If the risk of breast cancer among Dutch women could be reduced to that of Spanish women, nearly 60 new cases in every 100,000 women could be avoided each year. Less marked, but still important, variations are apparent when mortality rates from breast cancer are compared. In this comparison, Danish women had the highest and Greek women the lowest mortality rates. In general, there is a trend that more women living in northern Europe develop breast cancer than those living in southern Europe.

These figures need to be interpreted with care. When making comparisons by place (or time), it is worth asking whether the observed differences could be due to variations between groups in:

◆ how the disease was identified (ascertainment);

◆ how clinicians diagnosed and reported the disease (diagnosis);

◆ the structure of the populations being compared.

In the example (Fig. 3.2) the differences between countries may be explained, at least in part, by variations in how breast cancer was ascertained. For example, some countries have national screening programmes that aim to detect tumours at an early stage when treatment is usually easier. As a consequence, these countries may have higher incidence rates because they pick up small tumours that may be missed in countries without these screening services. There may also have been differences in what clinicians in each country diagnose as breast cancer. Cancer registers, upon which incidence data are based, vary in their completeness and accuracy both between and within countries. Some of the variation may be explained by differences between women living in the different countries in the numerous lifestyle, demographic, and socioeconomic factors that have been linked to breast cancer. At present, much interest is focused on dietary factors. Compared with their northern neighbours, southern Europeans tend to consume less fat and animal products, and more fruit and vegetables, dietary factors that have been associated with a reduced risk of breast cancer in some studies.

Perceptions depend upon where you look

Our perceptions about the relative size and importance of a particular health problem in society depend greatly on what information we use to assess the situation. Box 2 indicates some of the sources of information that are readily available to clinicians, managers, and researchers trying to assess whether health care is adequate, appropriate, effective, or cost-effective.

BOX 2 Some routinely available sources of data that give an epidemiological picture of society in the United Kingdom

- **Mortality data**—often given by cause of death, age, gender.
- **Hospital and clinical activity statistics**—these cover a variety of activities including acute inpatient and day case activity, admissions to mental hospitals, outpatient activity, maternity services, bed occupancy, and waiting times for planned appointments and admissions.
- **Reproductive health statistics**—includes information about number of births, miscarriages, and induced abortions, teenage pregnancy rates, use of family planning services, rates of maternal, neonatal, and infant deaths, and congenital abnormality rates.
- **Infectious disease statistics**—for example, rates of notifiable diseases, sexually transmitted diseases, HIV and AIDS.
- **Cancer statistics**—compiled nationally from cancer registries around the country giving incidence and mortality rates by site, gender, and age.
- **Accident statistics**—includes accident-related deaths and emergency hospital admissions by type and cause of accident.
- **Morbidity statistics from general practice**—much information comes from large intermittent one-year studies of patterns of consulting with general practitioners or practice nurses in a sample of practices in England and Wales.

BOX 2 Continued

One such study was conducted in 1990/91. Some practices also supply information on a regular basis to centralized databases, which make the data available for monitoring or research purposes.

♦ **The Health Survey of England** and the **Health Survey of Scotland**—separate annual health interview and physical examination surveys of a random sample of the general population. Different clinical areas are chosen each year for particular emphasis. These surveys also collect information about lifestyle such as smoking and drinking habits, physical activity, and diet.

♦ **General Household Survey**—an annual household survey of about 17,000 randomly chosen individuals with core questions about general health and socio-economic conditions. Additional health-related questions are occasionally included.

♦ **Labour Force Survey**—surveys of the population eligible to work, which also collects information about reasons for work absence.

♦ **Department of Social Security statistics**—these give information on days of certified incapacity for incapacity and/or invalidity benefit.

♦ **Drug misuse databases**—the collection of anonymous data on new problem drug users seen by a range of services including general practice and specialist drug services.

♦ **Expenditure on different NHS services**—including prescription data at regional, practice, and individual doctor level.

Much of the available information describes patterns of use of different health services. Such data cannot provide a complete picture of symptoms, illness or disease occurring in society. Everyday observations, and numerous one-off studies, tell us that many symptoms and illnesses occur in the community without ever being presented to healthcare professionals (See Chapter 4).

It is helpful to have some idea of how common a particular symptom is, if only to understand what might happen if a new treatment becomes available. For example, at present most people who suffer from migraines deal with the problem on their own. The introduction of a new migraine treatment could result in many of these individuals with previously 'unmet need' presenting to their general practitioners (GP) for the new treatment. The shift of a health problem from the community to primary care can have huge implications for the organization of primary care and the NHS resources that GPs are responsible for. New drugs for the treatments of obesity, influenza and impotence are now available: conditions that were previously largely self-managed in the community.

A general practice perspective

Most people in the UK (about 80%) consult their GP or practice nurse at least once a year; many consult much more frequently. Consultation rates vary with age and gender, with higher consulting rates at both extremes of age and among females (Fig. 3.3). In 1996, females saw their GP on average six times and males four times. Overall there were an estimated 284 million consultations with GPs during 1996, resulting in about 500 million prescriptions dispensed.

Many consultations are for immunizations and other preventive services such as well-woman and well-man check-ups. If these are ignored, the most common category of disease responsible for general practice attendance is respiratory problems (Fig. 3.4). This is not surprising given the high prevalence of respiratory symptoms in the general population. Overall, about a third of all patients who consult at least once each year do so because of a respiratory problem. About half of these consultations are for minor respiratory conditions, mainly acute upper respiratory tract infections. Problems affecting the nervous system or sense organs (largely infections of the ear or eye), injury and poisoning, and musculoskeletal problems are other large constituents of practice workload. In about 15% of all consultations the presenting health problem cannot be given a specific diagnostic label; many of these consultations are for abdominal pain, cough, headache, or rash.

Summary figures such as those in Fig. 3.4 are useful for given a broad-brush picture of practice workload. There are, however, important differences in the

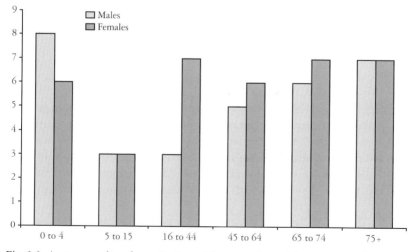

Fig. 3.3 Average number of consultations with a general practitioners per year, by age and gender, Great Britain 1996.

Source: OPCS (1996).

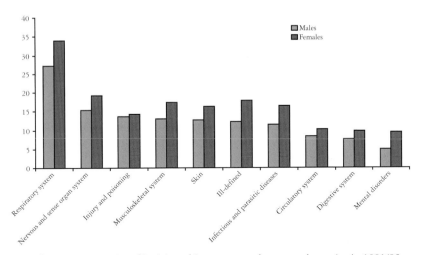

Fig. 3.4 Top 10 categories of health problems presented to general practice in 1991/92 by gender (percentage of patients consulting at least once). NB. Excludes consultations for preventative procedures such as immunizations.

Source: OPCS (1995).

use of general practice made by males and females at different ages. In young children, preventive procedures or generally minor conditions are the commonest reasons for being seen (Table 3.1). At the middle stage of life, respiratory infections, administrative matters, anxiety or depression, back pain, and sprains are the commonest reasons for men consulting. Women of a similar age have high consultation rates for pregnancy-related matters or contraception, respiratory infections, menstrual problems, anxiety or depression, and ill-defined symptoms. Attendances for family planning and pregnancy-related services account for a large part of the higher consulting rates among women aged 16–44 years (Table 3.1).

In older patients the effects of chronic, degenerative disease become apparent. Thus, in older male patients, the top five reasons for attendance are hypertension (high blood pressure), respiratory infections, chronic obstructive pulmonary disease or asthma, ill-defined symptoms, and ischaemic heart disease. Older females also attend often because of hypertension and respiratory infections, but their third most common reason is rheumatoid arthritis or osteoarthritic problems, followed by ill-defined problems, and anxiety or depression.

Information about age and gender differences is important for the planning of services that meet the needs of particular client groups within a practice. It also provides an indication about the impact (burden) that different diseases have for an individual and/or society, although other measures of burden are also needed. There are a number of alternative ways in which the burden

Table 3.1. Top five reasons for consulting with a doctor in general practice in 1991/92, at selected ages by gender

	0–4		25–44		65–74	
	Males	Females	Males	Females	Males	Females
1st	Acute respiratory infections	Acute respiratory infections	Acute respiratory infections	Pregnancy-related matters or contraceptions	Hypertension	Hypertension
2nd	Ear problems	Ear problems	Administrative issues, e.g. sick note	Acute respiratory infections	Acute respiratory infections	Acute respiratory infections
3rd	Immunizations	Immunizations	Anxiety or depression	Menstrual and related problems	Chronic obstructive pulmonary disease or asthma	Rheumatoid arthritis, osteoarthritis, and related problems
4th	Ill-defined symptoms	Ill-defined symptoms	Back problems	Anxiety or depression	Ill-defined symptoms	Ill-defined symptoms
5th	Dermatitis and related skin problems	Dermatitis and related skin problems	Joint sprains	Ill-defined symptoms	Ischaemic heart disease	Anxiety or depression

Source: OPCS, 1995.

associated with a particular disease can be evaluated. These include surveys that ask specifically about disability resulting from disease, and more general surveys that include questions about health problems affecting work, long-standing illness, or self-completed assessments of health status.

A hospital perspective

In 1997, there were about 8.5 million ordinary hospital admissions and 3 million day-case admissions throughout the UK. In addition, there were some 42 million out-patient attendances, of which about a quarter were new. This activity has increased dramatically during the past 20 years, especially with respect to day surgery which has increased more than six-fold because of recent surgical advances. The five most common operations performed in the NHS in Scotland in 1997 were cystoscopy, laparoscopy, lens operations (mostly cataract removal), varicose vein procedures, and inguinal or femoral hernia repairs.

Many patients admitted to hospital are at the severe end the spectrum of disease severity. It is not surprising, therefore, that hospital services account for just over half of all NHS expenditure, even though they deal with only a small fraction of ill-health occurring in our society. In terms of categories of disease, mental disorders account for about 17% of all NHS hospital expenditure, circulatory problems 11%, cancers 6%, respiratory disease 6%, injury and poisoning 6%, and musculoskeletal problems 6%. NHS expenditure is yet another way of assessing the burden of different diseases occurring in society, although we need to remember that individuals buy healthcare outside the NHS in the form of over-the-counter treatments, alternative medicine, etc.

A perspective from mortality data

Disease severity is also reflected in mortality data. Examination of mortality data reveals important age and gender differences, particularly when years of life lost are calculated, that is the total number of years of life lost by death under a certain age (normally less than 65 or 75 years). Determining the different causes of premature death is the first step towards action to prevent such events occurring in the future.

Overall, roughly half of all deaths in both men and women are due to circulatory disease, a third due to cancer and about 10% due to respiratory disease (Figs 3.5 and 3.6). When deaths under the age of 65 are examined, most deaths in men are due to injury and poisoning (mainly accidents and suicide), circulatory disease, or cancer. In women, cancers predominate, followed by circulatory disease and injury. When deaths under 75 years are examined the picture changes yet again. In men, circulatory disease becomes the leading cause of

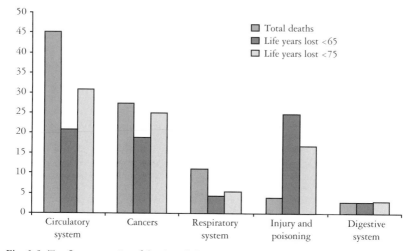

Fig. 3.5 Top five categories of death and their associated life-years lost in males, England 1991 (percentage of all deaths).

Source: NHS Executive (1996).

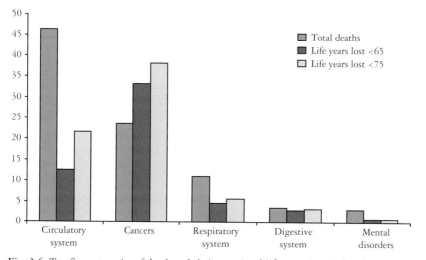

Fig. 3.6 Top five categories of death and their associated life-years lost in females, England 1991 (percentage of all deaths).

Source: NHS Executive (1996).

death, followed by cancer, injury, and poisoning. Among women, cancer continues to predominate (even more so), followed by circulatory disease, injury, and poisoning. Data such as these have led the government to set public health targets that seek to reduce the number of premature deaths occurring in the UK.

A constantly changing picture

As the profile of our society is constantly changing, so is the profile of disease affecting it. During this century, improved standards of living and important medical advances have contributed to reductions in the number of deaths due to infection, pregnancy, and congenital abnormalities. On the other hand, other diseases such as asthma, lung cancer, and diabetes have become more common. Within each disease group, major changes have occurred. For example, the number of women suffering from cancer of the stomach or ovary has declined, whereas the number developing lung cancer has increased dramatically. Within infectious disease, new organisms like HIV, campylobacter, and chlamydia have been discovered, while others like polio and measles have been virtually eradicated.

The last 50 years has seen an explosion of knowledge about risk factors associated with disease. This often leads to medical interventions to reduce the effects of these risk factors later in life. For instance, the screening for and treatment of raised blood pressure, greatly reduces an individual's risk of stroke or heart disease later in life. Some strategies to tackle high prevalence of risk factors in society require a wide range of professionals and organizations working together. Thus, strategies to reduce the number of people smoking requires the efforts of doctors, teachers, politicians, and health promotion staff among many others.

We need, therefore, to understand how the epidemiology of our society is changing if we are to make healthcare services responsive to need. In the not too distant future, we may have an even better understanding of the complex inter-relationship between the biological, genetic, environmental, and cultural factors that determine both the onset of disease, and its presentation to healthcare professionals. This knowledge will lead to the introduction of new screening services to prevent disease and improved targeting of interventions to treat established disease. Epidemiology will continue to guide the provision of appropriate, effective, and economical healthcare services in our society.

SUMMARY POINTS

- ◆ Epidemiology compares groups (study populations) to detect differences between them that might indicate the causes of an illness, the scope for prevention, or how to identify those at highest risk from disease(s).

- ◆ Comparisons usually involve calculating how often a particular event (or events) occurs in each group (the event rate) and measuring the characteristics of different groups (e.g. age, gender, ethnic origin, lifestyle) to see whether there is any possible connection between a characteristic and a disease. However, beware an association of this sort must not be assumed to be due to cause and effect.

SUMMARY POINTS Continued

♦ Common event rates include incidence, prevalence, and mortality rates.

♦ There is a large number of sources of routinely available data, which may be used for epidemiological purposes. These are principally data available from death certificates, hospital activities, registration of particular diseases, GP consultation data, and details of NHS prescriptions.

References and further reading

Beaglehole, R., Benita, R. and Kjellström, T. (2000). *Basic Epidemiology*. World Health Organization, Geneva.

Last, J.M. (2001). *A Dictionary of Epidemiology*, 4th edn. Oxford University Press, Oxford.

NHS Executive (1996). *Burdens of Disease*, a discussion document. DoH, London.

OPCS (1995). *Morbidity Statistics from General Practice*, Fourth Morbidity Survey 1991/92. HMSO, London.

OPCS (1996). *Living in Britain: results from the 1996 General Household Survey*. HMSO, London.

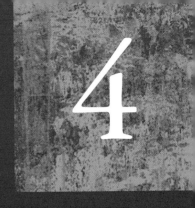

4

CHAPTER 4

How do we know we are healthy?

CHAPTER 4

How do we know we are healthy?

Defining health

The main thing is that I've still got my health.

'Health' is a much used, but less understood word. Most people recognize the importance of health, but would be hard-pushed to define what they mean by a statement such as the above. Health is a complex concept, which is perhaps easier to define by its absence than its presence. Despite this difficulty with precise definition, people usually know what they mean when they talk about their health. With a simple word they encompass a whole range of ideas, some of which could be easily pinpointed and others of which are more elusive. 'Health' can also mean different things to different people.

The word 'health' derives from the Old English word meaning 'wholeness'. It is most important to establish that 'health' properly refers to psychological and social well-being, and not just physical. This is particularly important in the community setting, where doctors are expected to treat illness in the context of the 'whole person', and his or her family and society roles. It can be argued that in most instances the individual is best placed to assess his or her own health. You know and feel more about your own psychological, social, and physical well-being than anyone else. You are that 'whole person'.

The task of all doctors is to find and 'treat' the psychological, the social, the environmental, *and* the physical disorders, and eventually improve the patient's overall quality of life. A primary task is to recognize the relative importance of each of these. For example, a young single mother, who is unable to sleep because her baby cries constantly, and because she is worried about lack of money and the threat of eviction from her house, is unlikely to have her quality of life improved significantly by the prescription of sleeping tablets. Conversely, people with serious physical disability can have great quality of life, and consider themselves to be healthy (see Chapter 16).

Medical versus lay perspectives

The way in which a doctor defines or conceives health may be different from that of his patient. This difference, if significant, may lead to difficulties and be detrimental to the care of that patient. Consider the following two cases:

CASE 1

A 55-year-old man is started on treatment for high blood pressure. This was detected 'opportunistically' (by chance, as part of a consultation for another matter) and warrants treatment to reduce his risk of having a stroke. However, high blood pressure produces no symptoms and will not be considered an illness by the man unless the implications are explained. Lack of proper explanation might cause a failure to take the prescribed medication and a resultant higher than necessary risk of serious illness.

CASE 2

A mother is extremely worried about her young child's high fever and vomiting, particularly as an outbreak of meningitis has received recent media publicity. On examination, her doctor is quickly able to attribute the problem to a simple virus infection, which will resolve spontaneously in a day or two. He tells her simply to give the child some paracetamol and fluids until the illness has gone. This is appropriate advice, but unless it is accompanied by strong re-assurance and a concerned attitude, with the opportunity to consult again should matters change, a major health issue, that of maternal anxiety, remains un-addressed.

In both these cases the doctor could be said to be acting appropriately on medical grounds, yet in each case there is clearly a problem. Definitions of health shared by patients and doctors would have avoided these problems. In Case 1 the man felt well and therefore did not recognize a health problem. In Case 2 the doctor found only a trivial problem, but left the mother with the belief that there was a serious problem.

Most people want to be healthy. For some people this is an important driver in their life, while for others it appears less important. However, if health is expanded beyond the physical dimension to include social indicators (such as belonging to a group) or psychological (such as the ability to have 'time for yourself'), we can see that even the habitual beer-drinking smoker might be actively in pursuit of a form of good health.

So what *is* health?

As doctors, your job will be to strive for the health of your patients, either on an individual or a community basis. Clearly, this would rarely involve a recommendation to start smoking. If we are to devote our careers to it surely we must know what we mean by 'health' right from the beginning.

When the National Health Service was formed in 1948, a stated goal was 'Health for all by the year 2000'. The premise was that if everyone had free access to health care, all illness in the country would be treated. The task of the NHS would be great at first, but become smaller as time progressed towards the end of the millennium. In fact, it is true that the task was great in 1948, but the workload has only increased since then. Why is this? Is the amount or of illness increasing? Is illness becoming more difficult to treat? Is the definition of illness or health changing?

It is unrealistic to expect a patient to come with a well thought-out definition of health or a typed summary of her own health beliefs. As professionals, though, we must be aware of some of the implications of the complexities and differences.

Consider these definitions of health (Collier *et al.* 1991):

1. Health is the absence of disease.

2. Health is a state of complete physical, mental, and social well-being (World Health Organization definition).

3. Health designates a process of adaptation—to changing environments, to growing up and ageing, to healing when damaged, to suffering, and to the peaceful expectation of death. Health embraces the future, and therefore includes anguish and the inner resources to live with it (Ivan Illich).

Which of these is the best definition? Is any of them complete? Each of them has limitations, which can be illustrated by consideration of the following cases:

- Mary Queen of Scots on the walk to her execution.
- A monk who has generalized weakness as a result of prolonged fasting.
- A farmer who lost a finger in an accident during his boyhood.
- A baby.

Which of these could be healthy by the above definitions? Each could be considered healthy by at least one definition, but none could by all definitions. We know which of them might be healthy and which might not (Table 4.1).

Table 4.1 The definition of health

Healthy?	Definition 1	Definition 2	Definition 3
Mary Queen of Scots	Yes	No	Possibly
Monk	Yes	No	Yes
Farmer	No	No	Yes
Baby	Yes	Yes	No

(Adapted from Collier *et al.* 1991)

A pragmatic definition

One useful way of considering health might be that aspect of being in which a deterioration leads to an individual wishing to seek medical advice. This recognizes a spectrum, rather than a dichotomy, and allows an understanding of health in relative terms, rather than absolute. It is a pragmatic definition, which excludes many episodes of ill health, but we might suppose includes all the important ones, in that, as doctors, we need not be interested in any of the exclusions. This falls down on two accounts.

First, there is enormous variability between individuals and societies in the threshold of symptoms beyond which medical advice is sought. This depends upon a large number of variables, including: personal attitudes towards and fears resulting from the symptoms, expectations of the family or society, and/or cultural background (see Chapter 5).

An individual's health beliefs (see also Chapter 13) are important. For example, if a young man believes that a persistent tickly cough is highly suggestive of lung cancer, he is likely to seek medical advice early in the course of the illness, even though this is an extremely unlikely diagnosis. If, however, an older man believes his cough of 3 months duration, accompanied by weight loss and haemoptysis (coughing up blood) represent simply a slight worsening of his 'normal' smoker's cough, he may not visit the doctor, and his lung cancer will remain undetected.

The following diagram, which is based on illness in the community, has been proposed (Fig. 4.1). It is a graphic illustration of the high frequency with which illness occurs in the adult population, and the relatively small proportion that is

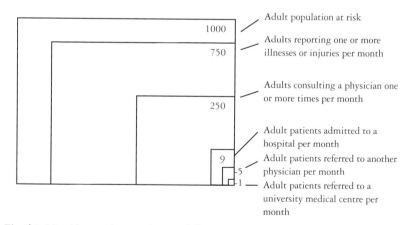

Fig. 4.1 Monthly prevalence estimates of illness in the community and the roles of physicians, hospitals and university medical centres in the provision of medical care (adults aged 16 years and over; White *et al.* 1961). Copyright © 1961 Massachusetts Medical Society, all rights reserved.

brought to a doctor. It is also of interest to note the very small proportion of illnesses that require specialist medical advice.

Secondly, this pragmatic definition would miss factors that we know affect health adversely. Part of a doctor's role is seen to be to inform patients of any health risk they may have and thereby to prevent illness in the future. This role drives cervical screening, which is the pre-symptomatic detection of cervical cancer; part of a woman's health care now includes having a cervical smear test. This role also makes the campaigns for reduction in smoking or unwanted pregnancies legitimate parts of the medical profession's duty.

Normality

'Normality' like 'health' is a word that is easy to use, but difficult to define and there may be overlap in our understanding of the two terms. We can define it in several ways, with several different terms of reference.

I Statistical

Statisticians have very precise definitions of normality. These are used frequently in discussions about health, the implication often being that significant deviation from normal defines illness. Figure 4.2 shows the birth weights of a hypothetical sample of babies.

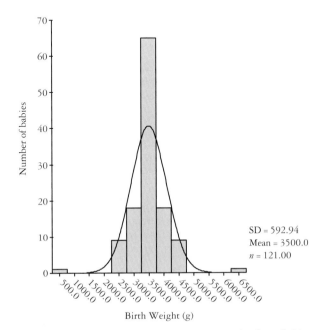

Fig. 4.2 Distribution of birth weights of a hypothetical sample of 121 babies.

This shows a mean, median, and modal birth weight of 3500 g, and an even distribution of other birth weights around this weight. The curve that is drawn over the bar chart is symmetrical and bell-shaped, representing a distribution of data known as a 'normal distribution'. A figure that can be calculated from the mean of the data is the standard deviation (SD). This is a measure of the spread of data about the mean and is 593 g in this case.

Where the values are distributed normally, as here, we note that around 66% of values lie within the range of the mean plus or minus the SD. We further note that around 95% of the values lie within the range of the mean ± 2 SD, and that around 99% lie within the range of the mean ± 3 SD. According to statistical convention, the range within which values are said to be 'normal' is often taken to be the mean plus or minus a multiple of the SD, and this multiple is commonly 2. This is useful in many cases in that it includes the vast majority of values, leaving out only those that fall at the extreme ends of the scale.

In our hypothetical data set, we find that this gives us a normal range of birth weights of 2314–4686 g. Anything outside this range could be classified as outside the normal range, and would include the values of 500, 2300, 4700, and 6500 g. Few obstetricians would argue with the first and the last of these, but what of the other two?

From population statistics to individuals

In reality, both 2300 and 4700 g can be 'normal' weights for a baby, and delivery of a baby of these weights will rarely give rise to concern. However, if a woman who has had three babies weighing around 2300 g then has one who weighs 4700 g, some concern would be expressed in case there was a serious reason for this sudden rise in birth weight. Conversely, a baby of 2300 g born to a woman who has had three babies weighing over 4700 g might be examined and observed in case there was a medical problem causing poor growth.

A similar picture could be painted for adult waist circumference, with which the 'normal' would be considerably greater in affluent Western societies than in societies where over-eating is less prevalent.

II Cultural

Another way of defining 'normal' is in cultural terms. Definitions here would tend to be less precise, but perhaps more important to individuals, and often dictated by current fashions and social pressures.

A typical example is body shape. It is easy to be led by magazines, advertising, and peers into thinking that a tall slim shape is the normal figure to have. It is equally easy to be led from this belief into one that says that any other shape is therefore abnormal, yet one only needs to stand on the corner of the high street for 2 minutes to notice the huge variety of body shapes and sizes in which members of our society present. Unfortunately, and despite this, many people devote considerable effort, money, and emotion to developing or preserving a fashionable figure. In many cases, this is unsuccessful, because the desired shape is unattainable with the given genetic make-up, or because of an inability to adhere to a particular rigorous diet and exercise programme. Failure often leads to feelings of guilt and loss of self-confidence, and the ramifications can be great. We see here the origins of serious conditions, such as anorexia or bulimia, but we also see the difficulties of imposing cultural 'norms' that are often arbitrary.

Another example is alcohol consumption. A normal level of drinking in one section of society will be unacceptable in another, and may bear little relation to the level defined as 'safe' by health professionals. At which point is drinking to be called abnormal, heavy, or indicative of alcoholism? Some groups tell us that more than 21 units of alcohol per week (1 unit $= \frac{1}{2}$ pint of beer, 1 glass of wine, 1 measure of spirits) for a man, or 14 units per week for a woman constitutes unsafe or heavy drinking. With this definition there will be many groups where the majority of members are 'alcoholic'. In these groups, little or no alcohol consumption will be abnormal. While such a level may be detrimental to physical health in the long term, abstinence, by leading to exclusion from the cultural norm of a group, may cause problems with other aspects of health. Conversely, if a man who was previously tee-total suddenly starts to drink 5 pints of beer every Friday and Saturday, a serious underlying reason may be present.

In each of these examples it becomes clear that defining or comparing with normal is not always useful by itself. With babies' birth weights, adults' waistlines, or dangerous alcohol consumption, it is far more important to know the background of the individual concerned and how the current situation relates to this.

III Perceived normality

'I know I am normal, but I am not so sure about anyone else.' There has been much philosophical debate over the nature of mental illness. One school of thought perceives mental illness as simply an extension of the 'normal' difference between individuals. The same might be true of physical illnesses. It is not clear at which point a loss of suppleness that could be described as 'normal', with age becomes an illness or 'arthritis'. This will presumably reflect individuals' perceptions, experiences and expectations.

The whole world's gone mad except thee and me—and tha's a bit queer!

IV Pathological

Finally, normality may be considered using the pathologist's frame of reference. When this doctor studies a biopsy specimen microscopically, she is often searching for 'abnormal' cells and would be happy to report only the presence of 'normal' ones. The implication, and it is usually correct here, is that normality is equivalent to health and abnormality to disease. This approach becomes dangerous, however, if it is applied uncritically in the consulting room. For example, a 'normal' rectal examination does not rule out rectal cancer and a 'normal' ultrasound scan in pregnancy does not exclude serious fetal abnormalities.

Just as with 'health', there is no single satisfactory definition of 'normality'. In different circumstances it might be more appropriate to apply statistical, cultural, perceptual, or pathological definitions. It is perhaps more important to recognize the potential problems with each of these than the correctness, when dealing with illness in the community.

SUMMARY POINTS

◆ 'Health' means different things to different people. Health is a very complex concept and examines different ways of viewing health.

◆ In particular, the lay view (of patients) may be quite different from the medical view (of doctors) and this is a potential source of much confusion in the consultation.

◆ Various definitions of health are analysed. None is perfect or all-embracing. One useful though imperfect working definition is 'that aspect of being in which a deterioration leads to an individual wishing to seek medical advice'.

◆ Definitions of health depend on individual's health beliefs and a concept of what is normal, in itself a very complex field. The chapter concludes with a detailed analysis of different concepts of 'normality'—the statistical, the cultural, the individual's perception, and pathological definitions.

References and further reading

Bland, M. (2000). *An Introduction to Medical Statistics*, 3rd edn. Oxford University Press, Oxford.

Collier, J.A.B., Longmore, J.M. & Harvey, J.H. (1991). *Oxford Handbook of Medical Specialties*, 3rd edn. Oxford University Press, Oxford.

White, K.L., Williams, F. & Greenberg, B.G. (1961). The ecology of medical care. *New England Journal of Medicine*, **265**, 885–892.

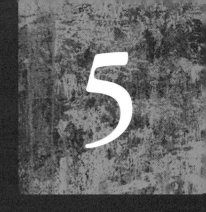

5

CHAPTER 5

What do we mean by illness?

CHAPTER 5
What do we mean by illness?

Introduction

In the previous chapter, we recognized that health is not an easily defined concept. What, though, about the other side of the coin? How do we know when we are ill or recognize illness in others? We saw that, in most cases, there were aspects of illness and health that were present in the same individual. We will also see that, in society, a substantial amount of illness is present at any one time. We now propose that health and illness are not mutually exclusive, i.e. one is not either healthy or ill. Rather health and illness are two parts of a spectrum; illness is part of normality and, consequently, illness is as difficult to define as health.

Illness and disease

There is an important sociological difference between these two terms that influences our dealings with patients. *Disease* implies an entity that we can isolate and eliminate; in many cases, diseases are merely collections of symptoms and clinical findings assembled for the convenience of the medical profession and the patient. This has advantages in aiding treatment and prognosis, but it may encourage consideration of the physical disease at the expense of considering the patient. If no disease is found, the disease-bound outlook may dismiss symptoms as being 'in the mind', neurotic, or irrelevant. However, symptoms do not arise without some reason and the reasons may be complex. *Illness* exists independently of identifiable specific symptoms and signs, and includes the patient's sensations and feelings, disabilities, discomforts attitudes, and the effects of the symptoms on activities and relationships. Symptoms are not confined to physical effects.

> Disease is diagnosed.
> Illness is experienced.

Patients may present to the doctor with a disease and no illness, or vice versa. High blood pressure, because of the known resulting increased risk of strokes, has been labelled a disease (hypertension), yet usually causes no symptoms and 'sufferers' do not experience illness. On the other hand, there are many who present with symptoms of chronic fatigue and lethargy in whom no diagnosis is possible and no disease tag conferred. In fact, no disease specific diagnosis is possible in up to

50% of patients who attend their GP, as the symptoms do not conform to a recognized disease pattern.

Acute and chronic illness

Simply, acute illness is short-term or the short-term stages of an illness; chronic illness is long-term. Many illnesses, such as most infections, are always acute and some, such as Parkinson's disease, are always chronic. Other conditions can have acute and chronic stages. Many chronic diseases, such as chronic bronchitis, are complicated by periodic acute exacerbations. There is no temporal dividing line between acute and chronic illness, although sometimes, as in the case of pain, an arbitrary one is imposed (3 months). It is probably an attitudinal, rather than a temporal change, in that management of acute illness tends to focus on cause and cure, while management of chronic disease tends to focus on limitation of effects, dealing with these, and maximizing patients' potential quality of life.

Since the instigation of the NHS in 1948 in the UK there has been a steady shift of the pattern of illness treated in the community, from acute to chronic. This has been the result of huge advances in treatments, such as antibiotics, and a greater life expectancy such that degenerative diseases (such as cancer and arthritis) have assumed a greater prominence.

Health and illness: a spectrum rather than a dichotomy

Most people have regular and irregular spells of illness. Most of us expect to get a cold or 'flu once or twice a year; nearly every reader will have had at least one of the childhood diseases (e.g. chicken pox or rubella), most adolescents in the industrialized world experience sports injuries, and many women experience period pains. A substantial number of people wear glasses or contact lenses, but somehow we do not regard most of these people as being ill or disabled. Most people in the industrialized world will have been hospitalized for some kind of operation. In other words, being ill is part of life. It is normal!

We need to consider illness and disease by age, within the context of normality. Thus, babies, toddlers, middle-aged men, and women over 80 show different patterns of illness, and the same disease might manifest itself in different ways or have a greater or lesser influence across the age ranges. Failing sight would cause considerable concern in a 20-year-old, but may pass unremarked upon in the later stages of life. These patterns have been explored in Chapter 3. An understanding of a patient's background and expectations will assist us in addressing their symptoms. However, just because an illness is 'normal' does not mean that we can ignore it. Chapter 11 discusses the dangers of age-based prejudice in addressing symptoms.

The influence of culture

Factors inherent within a given culture are also likely to influence deeply the perception and definition of illness, and any consequent actions. In the Old Testament of the Bible, disease was often seen as a curse from God or a punishment for sin. In the New Testament, mental illness was seen as the influence of or occupation by demons. In some cultures, disease has magical or mystical qualities, perhaps the result of a spell or the influence of the moon (lunacy). In each of these cases attempts at cures followed from the specific views of 'aetiology', e.g. spiritual or magical. In modern Western culture we tend towards a biophysical view of illness, such that cures are very often drug-based, even where this is inappropriate (for example, antibiotics for viral sore throats). Perhaps somewhere in between is most appropriate.

Similar to other epidemic diseases Acquired Immune Deficiency Syndrome (AIDS), caused by the Human Immunodeficiency Virus (HIV), is surrounded by a bizarre set of beliefs. Infectious diseases always inspire fears of easy contagion, such as the plague (*Yersinia pestis*), syphilis, and smallpox. Like most plagues, AIDS is a scourge of poor people worldwide. AIDS has caused uncertainty and fear because the disease is strongly associated with taboos—sex, sexuality, sexually transmitted diseases, mind-altering/illegal drugs, death, and dying. Widespread fear of AIDS *and* AIDS sufferers still exists in our society, even though it is proven that AIDS is not communicable through normal social contact. One study (Walkey *et al.* 1990) showed that AIDS patients were deemed more 'dangerous, dirty, foolish and worthless' in comparison to descriptions of cancer or coronary heart patients. In addition, victims tend to be labelled as either 'guilty' (through drug-use or sexual promiscuity) or 'innocent' (through infected blood products or babies born to infected mothers).

Certain cultural beliefs are held in modern society despite strong evidence to the contrary. For example, many (or most) people persist in the view that exposure to rain will precipitate pneumonia or a 'chill', or that leaving the house (or even the bed) when suffering with a cold will exacerbate that illness. Both of these constitute pure mythology, yet are remarkably prevalent. Other lay beliefs (or 'old wives' tales') include such worthy maxims as 'feed a cold and starve a fever'.

Health and illness in the community

Health and illness in the community have been studied in a number of ways. Some surveys have asked about the presence of particular symptoms, while others have enquired about a history of specific diagnoses. Some studies have involved the physical examination of people and used the presence of risk factors, such as high blood pressure or obesity as surrogate indicators of disease.

Community surveys of symptoms find a high level of occurrence of symptoms. In 1972, interviewers asked approximately 1300 Glaswegians whether they or their children had experienced a wide range of physical or mental symptoms in the previous 2 weeks. Nearly all of the participants (86%) had had at least one physical symptom, with an average of 4.3 and a maximum of 25. Just over half of all adults reported having at least one mental symptom, with an average of 1.1 per adult and a maximum of seven. Respiratory symptoms were the most common physical symptoms, followed by feeling tired and headaches (Fig. 5.1). Feelings of low spirits and anxiousness were the most common mental symptoms (Fig. 5.2; Hannay 1979).

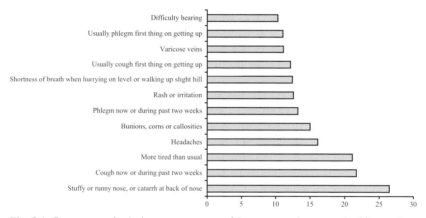

Fig. 5.1 Commonest physical symptoms reported in a community survey in Glasgow in 1972: 2-week prevalence (percentage of all participants of all ages).
Source: Hannay (1979).

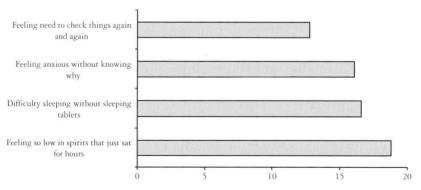

Fig. 5.2 Commonest mental symptoms reported in a community survey: 2-week prevalence (percentage of all adult participants).
Source: Hannay (1979).

The participants considered most of the symptoms to be non-severe or non-serious. The study showed, however, that it would be wrong to assume that everyone with symptoms or signs of serious disease will seek medical help. About a quarter of participants who reported a medical symptom that they considered to be severe or serious did not seek professional help. This figure contrasts with 11% of participants with non-severe or non-serious symptoms who sought professional help. In general, people seem more willing to report physical symptoms than mental symptoms.

Clearly, the findings of surveys such as the Glaswegian one depend greatly on what exactly is asked. They are also highly dependent on the structure of the population being studied. Age, cultural gender, socio-economic circumstances, past medical history, and personal characteristics are among the numerous factors that influence (by varying degrees) both the reported prevalence of symptoms and decisions about whether to seek help. These are discussed in Chapter 3, and also in Chapters 7 and 10.

Seeking medical advice

Most health care in Britain today consists of self-medication—drugs bought over the counter (i.e. without a medical prescription), traditional remedies, and alternative medicine. These figures (and Fig. 4.1 in Chapter 4) confirm that much illness remains unattended for some reason. They also suggest that illness requiring (or instigating the quest for) medical attention is a normal part of Western adult life. They may even suggest that absence of any symptoms or injury is almost abnormal (but that these are serious in relatively few cases). We know that different groups of people attend the doctor with differing frequencies. Women from all social classes, for example, consult the doctor more often than men do, while the very young and very old are also frequent attenders. There are likely to be several reasons for this, which should be explored and are only partly explained by incidence of biophysical pathologies.

Factors affecting the desire for treatment

Within social sub-groups different consultation rates can be seen. Part of this is related to people's view of their illness and their thresholds in different circumstances. The same set of symptoms may be regarded differently and lead to different behaviour in two individuals. Why should this be? There are often 'triggers' for the seeking of medical advice or other factors affecting the desire for professional advice. These are not directly related to the severity of symptoms, nor do they necessarily relate to stoicism.

> ### BOX 1 Factors affecting the desire to seek professional medical advice
>
> 1. A crisis, such as bereavement or redundancy, such that a person's normal coping mechanisms are disrupted.
> 2. Symptoms that are felt to interfere with work, physical activity, or social or personal relationships.
> 3. Pressure or advice from others (friends, family, employers) to seek help or care.
> 4. Symptoms that are externally visible (e.g. skin conditions).
> 5. Symptoms that conform to a pattern recognizable from previous experience (e.g. an early recurrence of depression).
> 6. Symptoms that are perceived to signify serious disease.
> 7. Cultural and social background and health beliefs.
> 8. Anxiety (which may expedite or delay consultation).
> 9. Other factors making consultation difficult, such as surgery hours, availability of child care, or embarrassment.
>
> (Zola 1973; Mechanic 1968)

It becomes clear, therefore, that a person's view of any set of symptoms is subject to multiple influences that will vary enormously between and within individuals. Psychological and sociological models are therefore important, not only in explaining frequency of consultation, but also in managing individual people. In these models, it is proposed that, unless a person's reasons for the holding of his or her perspective are addressed, it is unlikely that treatment or advice will be successful in reaching the desired end. An example is the patient who attends with chronic backache in the belief that this pain signifies cancer. Even though there is a benign explanation for his pain, if this belief is not aired and addressed he may continue to have an inappropriate view of his symptoms, and suffer continued anxiety, which is likely to make his symptoms worse and increase his attendance rate.

Lay referral

Before or in addition to attendance at a doctor is a system that has been described as 'lay referral', where symptoms or findings are discussed or presented to people such as families, friends, and colleagues. Here, symptoms may be 'confirmed', explained, or exaggerated, and the subsequent perception affected. For example, in pregnancy, women who may be experiencing alarming symptoms for the first time, often seek the advice of their mothers or of friends who have been pregnant. Common symptoms of pregnancy, such as abdominal discomfort, can thus be explained in a variety of ways, depending on the experiences of the women who have been 'consulted'. The relationship between this advice and conventional medical belief may be significant or minimal, but either way its effect on the perception of the pregnancy will influence the decision to consult a doctor or midwife. Obviously, lay referral may either increase or decrease consultation tendencies in particular instances, but some research has shown that there may be around 11 'lay consultations' for every medical consultation.

Other influences

Social situations can play a role in defining illnesses. Workers whose pay is reduced by sickness absence are probably less likely to consult during illness than those whose pay remains unaffected. This can lead to an under-reporting on the one hand and an over-enthusiastic rate of reporting on the other! Formerly, employers could insist that all sickness absence be confirmed by a certificate issued by a doctor. This led to such a high rate of consultation for minor illness that a system of self-certification for the first week of illness was introduced. Nonetheless, employers' demands are still influential in the seeking of medical advice.

The sick role

People often define illness in lay terms as an inability to do something, whether this is writing an essay, attending the nightclub or making a cup of tea. However, if this inability to do things, to fulfil social obligations, lasts beyond a certain time, the 'ill' person is expected to contact a medical practitioner. One of the tasks of the medical practitioner is to verify the presence of illness and then sanction its presence. This process makes the ill person an 'official' patient with a 'sick role'. This concept was first introduced in the 1950s, when it was seen essentially as a temporary and undesirable role.

Patients are 'allocated' a sick role by their society (family, friends, colleagues). This is a pattern of expectations regarding how an ill person should behave. The sick role essentially 'prescribes' what rights sick persons can claim and what obligations they should discharge. In general, society does not blame the sick for their illness, because they do not choose to be sick. They are not regarded as being responsible for their illness. Therefore, they have the right to be taken care of by others. However, there may be exceptions, such as AIDS or, increasingly, 'smoking-related' diseases. 'Playing' the sick role gives the individual the right to be exempted from certain social duties: they should not be forced to go to work; they should be excused from participation in many daily chores; students should be allowed to miss an exam and take it later. However, the sick have duties too, according to those studying the sick role. They are obliged to get well if they can. The sick should not use the illness to take advantage of others' love, concern, sympathy, and care for them; neither should they shirk their work and social responsibilities. The sick are expected to 'work' towards getting better, through the process of seeking professional medical help, and to co-operate with prescribed treatment.

The doctor–patient roles and relationships

The social construction of the consultation process is important, influencing rates of attendance and perceptions of illness. Most doctors recognize that most consultations with patients are not simply a process whereby experts give advice to lay people after the latter have described their problems. More often than not the consultation is a negotiation process between the patient, who is expert on his or her own health and life, and the doctor, who is expert on medical conditions.

The relationship between the doctor and the patient is of utmost importance, and must be seen as an interaction, with each party influencing both the other and the process of consultation. Respective roles may be seen differently by different people, doctors, and patients. These factors are probably *at least* as important in diagnosis and therapy as scientific knowledge and drugs are. The doctor–patient relationship is therefore important in influencing perception of illness and is determined by many factors, including the age, gender, ethnic and social background, and personality of the patient and of the doctor.

The impact of illness

The effects of illness are not uni-dimensional. Every episode, even of the simplest illness, affects the patient's physical, psychological, and social milieus. The effect may also be economic if earning capacity is affected, or spiritual. Furthermore, the impact extends beyond the individual patient, with implications for carers, family, colleagues, and sometimes society as a whole. For these reasons, severity of illness is a relative measure and illness that would be mild for one person is more significant for another. Any illness that requires a self-employed patient to take sick leave will be perceived as severe. A 24-h episode of sickness and diarrhoea will be considered severe by the full-time mother of three young children, yet classed as minor by her physician. Any epileptic seizure has huge implications on employment and driving potential, and may thus have significant impact even several years after the last seizure. On the other hand, a patient with 'severe' heart disease may adjust his lifestyle to one of relative immobility, perhaps subconsciously, and not consider his illness significantly limiting or disabling. The spectrum of illness is complex.

SUMMARY POINTS

- ◆ 'Illness' and 'Disease' are separate, although related concepts. A patient may have a disease, but no illness (and vice versa). Disease is diagnosed, whilst illness is experienced.

- ◆ There is no exact cut-off between being 'well' and being 'ill'. We are all on a spectrum of health/illness. Being ill is a normal part of life!

- ◆ Management of acute illness tends to focus on cause and cure, whilst management of chronic illness focuses on limitation of damage and on maximizing the patients potential quality of life.

- ◆ Cultural beliefs have an important influence on perception of illness. Even in modern society, 'old wives' tales' abound and persist.

- ◆ Doctors need to know about 'patient pathways'. How do people decide that they are ill and how do they come to seek medical advice?

- ◆ The nature of the doctor–patient relationship also influences lay and professional perception of illness, and treatment of this.

References and further reading

Hannay, D.R. (1979). *The Symptoms Iceberg*. Routledge & Kegan Paul, London.

Mechanic, D. (1968). *Medical Sociology*. Free Press, London.

Porter, M., Alder, B., Abraham, C. (1999). *Psychology and Sociology Applied to Medicine: An Illustrated Colour Text*. Churchill Livingston, Edinburgh.

Walkey, F.H., Taylor, A.T.J. & Green, D.E. (1990). Attitudes to AIDS: a comparative analysis of a new and negative stereotype, *Social Science and Medicine*, **30**, 549–552.

Zola, I. (1973). Pathways to the doctor, *Social Science and Medicine*, 7, 677–689.

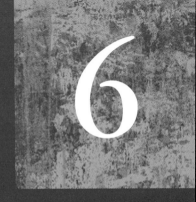

6

CHAPTER 6

Introduction: Influences on Health

CHAPTER 6
Introduction: Influences on Health

The first five chapters have provided an overview of health and illness in society. This overview outlined societal factors, such as the place of medicine in the community, the general influence of society on health and illness, the epidemiology of disease in our society, and personal factors, such as our own perceptions of being healthy and being ill.

The following five chapters provide a more detailed analysis of the different social and psychological factors, which influence health status. Chapter 7 addresses the range of social factors that influence people's health, such as gender, socio-economic status, ethnicity, and lifestyle. Chapter 8 looks at economic and political factors. Chapter 9 considers the environmental aspects, including biological, physical, and chemical influences on health. It is recognized that some also see psychosocial factors as part of the environmental factors influencing health and illness, but we feel these factors need to be addressed separately (see also Chapter 7). Chapter 10 considers the psychological factors that affect individuals' health. This chapter outlines the mental processes and ways humans deal with stress, through defence or coping mechanisms. Chapter 11 'Influence of age on health' addresses a main underlying influence on our health. This chapter also covers issues related to society's reaction to ageing, in terms of discrimination in the form of ageism. A more applied way of looking at behaviour and especially behavioural change can also be found in Chapter 13 'Health promotion'.

Being healthy: choice or determination?

There is a constant debate whether being healthy is a choice based on decisions taken by individuals regarding lifestyle and behaviour, or whether being healthy is determined by external factors, such as, for example, one's genes, social class, ethnic background, and/or personality. Few people argue the extreme views, i.e. that it is all due to choice or all determined. However, many argue about the degree of choice or the degree of determination in people's health. Is the state of one's health largely due to individual choices or is it largely due to social, economic, environmental, etc., factors?

These arguments are not purely philosophical or only of interest to academics. The definition of the issue has an influence on the way one tries to solve the health problem. For example, if one sees illegal drug use purely or largely as an individual choice, one would try to find a solution that involves getting (potential) drug misusers to make different choices. This could include health education interventions to warn drug misusers of the dangers and side-effects of drug use, but also prison sentences to make them think twice the next time they are in a position where they have to decide about using illegal substances. However, if one sees drug misuse largely as determined by external factors, such as unemployment, poor housing, lack of opportunities in life, etc., one would try to find different solutions to problem drug use. The latter approach might include skill training for drug misusers, creating jobs and/or improving council house estates.

Health: multidimensional?

Although this textbook highlights the different influences on health in different chapters, we would like to remind the reader that many of these factors are inter-related. For example, environmental factors such as chemicals might have a greater influence on some socio-economic groups than others, because lower socio-economics groups are more likely to work on the shop floor and come into contact with dangerous chemicals. Another example might be lifestyle factors and ethnicity. Diet, alcohol consumption, and smoking, for example, differ considerably between different ethnic groups. Thus, although we have presented the different factors influencing health in different chapters for clarity we stress that more often than not several factors together influence our health at any one time.

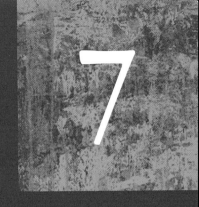

7

CHAPTER 7

Social influences on health

CHAPTER 7
Social influences on health

Introduction

Previous chapters have already demonstrated that social factors can have a very strong influence on the health of an individual, as well as that of a whole community. This chapter highlights this from a structural, sociological point of view, examining the main ways in which industrial societies are sub-divided. These include socio-economic factors, gender, ethnicity, and lifestyles.

Socio-economic factors

The idea that groups in society have different wealth, status, power, and privileges based on their economic position in society has a long history. Aristotle, for example, noted that:

> in all states there are three elements: one class is very rich, another very poor, and a third is mean.

Social class is a form of social stratification (literally layering of society). We are all familiar with the notion of a society divided up into 'working class', 'middle class', and 'upper class'. These different social strata have different chances and opportunities in life. This inequality between groups of people can also be observed in people's health experience. Thus, people in the top layer tend to have better chances in life than people in the bottom layer. For example, they live longer (lower mortality rates), are less likely to get a whole range of diseases (lower morbidity rates), are more likely to seek medical help early, are more likely to change lifestyle in response to health promotion interventions, and so on.

Definitions

Terms such as 'upper social class' have a precise academic definition. However, they are also part of our everyday language and have a common sense meaning. What constitutes a social class might vary between different countries, cultures, and societies. Furthermore, the definition of social class and/or its constitution has varied over time. Table 7.1 gives the most common occupational classification currently in use and as used in Britain since the 1911 Census (with minor variation over time).

Chapter 8 outlines some of the economic and political influences on health at an international and natural level. National economic factors influence total

Table 7.1 Social class in Britain in the early years of the twenty-first century

Social class	Definition	Examples of occupations
I	Professionals	Doctors, lawyers
II	Managerial and technical occupations	Company owners, managers, nurses
III (a)	Skilled occupations: non-manual	Sales workers, corner shop owners
III (b)	Skilled occupations: manual	Supervisors, technicians
IV	Partly skilled occupations	Farm and factory workers
V	Unskilled occupations	Porters, labourers

income available in a country. However, this chapter focuses more on division between groups within a society.

Numerous studies have indicated that there is a difference in life chances between social classes.

EXAMPLE 1 The sinking of the Titanic and survival of female passengers by social class

The point that one's social class determines survival rates was made clearly in 1912 at the time of the sinking of the Titanic.

The official casualty list showed that only 4 first-class passengers (3 voluntarily chose to stay on the ship) of a total of 143 were lost. Among the second-class passengers, 15 of 93 females drowned; and among the third-class, 81 of 179 female passengers went down with the ship. (Lord 1955)

The Black Report

One of the main recent overviews in the field of health and inequality in Britain was the 1980 *Black Report* (Townsend & Davidson, 1982). This listed four possible explanations for the differences between social class and health. These four explanations—artefact, materialistic, social selection, and cultural/behavioural—are summarized below.

Artefact

One possible explanation is that the observed differences between social classes are not real, but due to the way we conduct our measurements, i.e. compile the statistics. For example, establishing a specialist health clinic in a particular community, which picks up more cases of a disease than a standard clinic, would lead to biased reporting and, therefore, inflate disease rate statistics for that community. The failure of health inequalities to diminish is explained by the reduction of the proportion of people in the poorest occupation classes. The implication of this argument is that those who are upwardly mobile have a better health than those who remain.

Materialistic

The overall material resources available to different groups of people could also influence their health status. Lack of material resources stems from poverty, including being in low-paid work or unemployed, and is compounded by poor housing, poor working conditions (both physical and mental), poor social environment, lack of transport, and poor education. There is considerable evidence that as income increases the risk of mortality falls at a declining rate. In other words, an increase in income reduces the risk of mortality by a smaller amount for someone with a high income than for someone with a low income. A possible explanation for the factors at work is that the more income one earns the better food one can buy, the safer car one can drive, the better house one can afford, or the longer holidays one can book.

Social selection

This explanation centres on the notion that a 'natural' selection takes place, whereby the weaker, less healthy people end up in the lower social classes. For example, people who are ill for a long time might lose their jobs and experience what is called 'downward social mobility'. They might have to take less demanding jobs, because of their poor health and, consequently, they end up in a lower social class. The general consensus is that health selection does not occur to a sufficient extent to explain major health variation.

Cultural/behavioural explanations

The fourth explanation for health inequality in the Black report is centred round notions of culture and behaviour. Culture is a human creation, which includes codes of behaviour, dress, language, rituals, and systems of beliefs. People in different social classes behave differently and have different expectations—they have different lifestyles. For example, people in the lower social classes are more likely to smoke cigarettes and, therefore, are more likely to end up with smoking-related diseases. The lifestyle concept is a hotly debated topic. Some argue that it is simply a different way of approaching socioeconomic differences; others argue that lifestyles involve a certain element of choice in presenting the 'self'. Doctors can be involved in helping to change lifestyles, e.g. advising patients on doing more exercise or running smoking cessation classes. However, they cannot *effect* a change—this must be the result of independent choice and action by an individual.

The link between life chances and social class is more complicated than the seemingly straightforward link between health and wealth/income (or occupation or education level). There is often an additional link between the common beliefs in certain social classes, and the levels of health and illness.

One of the best pieces of research into lay aetiology was conducted in Aberdeen by Blaxter & Paterson (1982). They sought to clarify why those who most need medical services tend to use them least. This phenomenon 'the inverse care law' was first formally observed by a Welsh GP, Dr Julian Tudor-Hart (1971), in careful studies of his practice population The prior hypothesis was that perceptions of health in poor socio-economic conditions might create attitudes of apathy towards health care. Moreover, they assumed that these attitudes were transmitted through generations, especially through the female members of the family. A detailed study of the beliefs held by working-class mothers and grandmothers living in Aberdeen led to the conclusion that there were, indeed, similarities between the viewpoints of the two generations. However, these similarities were likely to be based on a common source, namely the social disadvantage itself that befalls both of the generations.

Social and cultural factors may also influence the process and outcome of the consultation, though these may be conscious or unconscious and may be advantageous or detrimental. The Black Report (Townsend & Davidson 1982) showed that illness is greatest in prevalence and seriousness among members of socio-economic group V (most deprived), yet rates of referral to hospital specialists are greatest among the most affluent socio-economic group I. Furthermore, the average duration of consultation increases from group V to group I.

Some argue that it is not simply the absolute income levels that determine people's life chances, but also the distribution of income (i.e. relative income or the 'rich-poor divide'). The proponents of this view link the national income distribution of a country to levels of inequality in health. Very large socio-economic differences between groups in society, they argue, can have a damaging effect on the overall health of a nation, regardless of the level of income. These large differences lead to a decrease in social cohesion in a society. A greater inequality (i.e. 'relative poverty') is associated with higher population mortality and this relationship persists even when account is taken of the average income of the population. Recent evidence appears to support this view (Wilkinson 1996).

Gender

There are differences between women and men in health status and uptake of health care. Men have a higher mortality at every age and women have a higher morbidity. For example, men are more likely to commit suicide than women, as illustrated in Table 7.2.

Table 7.2 Suicides and self inflicted injury, Scotland 1998

	Numbers	Rate per 100,000
Female	163	6.18
Male	486	19.56

Source: Registrar General (1999).

Women are known to consult the doctor more frequently than men. This can be explained partly by illnesses exclusive to or predominant among women, reproductive and contraceptive issues, and opportunities provided by coincident attendance with children. There is also a part to be played by factors such as the higher rate of full-time employment among men than women, such that men have less chance to attend a daytime surgery. A feminist view is that the medical profession is male-dominated and geared towards a patriarchal subjection of women to the system, which includes control of fertility, and the assumption that women's main role is in home-provision and child-care. An alternative view is that the system actually favours women, in that the nature of the doctor–patient relationship makes it harder for men to admit to certain symptoms, such as sexual dysfunction or depression, and the timing of surgeries is less likely to enable men to attend.

Ethnicity

Britain is a multicultural society. Its population originated in many different parts of the world, including Continental Europe, Ireland, Asia, the West Indies, and Africa. We use the term 'ethnicity', which is a broader concept than 'race', to analyse this diversity. Ethnicity includes social and cultural influences, as well as genetic factors. These issues again have an influence on the chances of staying healthy and falling ill, as well as on help seeking behaviour.

Research indicates that the lower socio-economic status of many ethnic minority groups has a large influence on health inequalities. For example, higher morbidity rates are found for all diseases in lower socio-economic groups; however, ethnic minority lower socio-economic groups have consistently higher morbidity rates for diseases such as coronary heart disease, diabetes, and hypertension than their white counterparts. But differences in the social experience of ethnic minority groups cannot be reduced to socio-economic factors alone—culture and race also need to be considered. Not all ethnic minorities are the same. There is evidence in Britain, for example, that on average those of Bangladeshi or Pakistani descent fall into lower socio-economic groupings than those from Afro-Caribbean descent. These differences also affect the chances of falling ill or dying.

Ethnicity includes communication issues. For example, elderly people who came to Britain at a later age might not be able to speak English well. Ethnic factors can also have an influence on a range of lifestyle issues such as diet, alcohol use, smoking and exercise, but also on more general health beliefs and health seeking behaviour. We have to be very careful not to use stereotypes of ethnic minorities and assume that everyone in a particular ethnic group acts in the same or a similar way.

Conclusions

There are real measurable differences in the life chances of different groups in society. There is agreement that morbidity and mortality rates differ between different groups in our society, for example between men and women, or between Britain's white majority and many of its ethnic minority groups, or between lower and higher social classes. Less agreement exists about the reasons for these differences. We suggest that materialist and lifestyle factors are more likely to explain these differences than the 'artefact' or the 'social selection' explanations. However, it is likely that the explanations for health variation are not simply uni-dimensional, but that these are complex and inter-related. What does this mean for medical students and doctors? It is important to note that beliefs about health and illness, and health-related behaviours are rooted in the wider context of people's lives. Sensitivity to the background of individual patients is important for doctors. However, being aware of the social, cultural, and ethnic background of your patients should not lead to stereotyping or attributing everything to such factors.

SUMMARY POINTS

- Society can be divided into six occupation-based social classes. These have close parallels with levels of income, but have other discrete differences.

- In general, rich people have better chances in life than poor people. They live longer, are less likely to contract disease, make better use of health-care systems, and are more likely to adapt healthy lifestyles.

- In the UK, the Black Report listed four possible explanations for this phenomenon—artefact, materialistic, social selection, and cultural/behavioural. These explanations are detailed in this chapter, but the best explanations are thought to be materialistic (i.e. differences in wealth) and lifestyle/cultural.

- Gender differences are a particular case, where it is thought that special factors have operated for women as opposed to men.

- Ethnicity is another particular example, where minority groups may experience health deprivation.

- Health workers can redress the balance by positive awareness and discrimination in favour of deprived groups.

References and further reading

Blaxter, M. & Paterson, E. (1982). *Mothers and Daughters: a three-generational study of health attitudes and behaviour*. Heinemann, London.

Lord, W.A. (1955). *Night to Remember*. New York: Henry Holt. Quoted In: Antonovsky, A. (1967). Social class, life expectancy and overall mortality. *Millbank Memorial Fund Quarterly*, **XLV**, 31–73.

Registrar General (1999). *Annual Report of the Registrar General of Births, Deaths and Marriages for Scotland 1998*. Registrar General Office for Scotland, Edinburgh.

Townsend, P. & Davidson, N. (eds) (1982). *Inequalities in Health: The Black Report*. Penguin, Harmondsworth.

Tudor Hart, J. (1971). The inverse care law. *Lancet*, i, 405–412.

Wilkinson, R.G. (1996). *Unhealthy Societies*. Routledge, London.

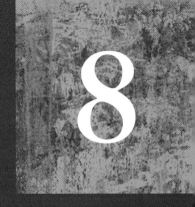

8

CHAPTER 8

Economic and political influences on health

CHAPTER 8

Economic and political influences on health

Introduction

Some of the factors that influence health operate at an individual level, while others operate at a society level, and some at both an individual and a society level, such as environmental or social factors. In this chapter we will address influences that are largely at a society level. The understanding of the distinction between the levels is important with regard to who has potential control of these influences on the health of both individuals and communities.

This chapter deals with economic and political influences on health, as well as their influences on health care provision. Economics is the discipline that studies the use of scarce resources, while politics deals with organization and government of communities. Political influence on health can work through economic controls, as well as through policies, legislation, information, and education.

Global economic influences on health

Chapter 7 described the socio-economic inequalities that affect the health of individuals. Table 8.1 gives a measure of wealth, the Gross National Product (GNP) *per capita*, for a range of developing and developed economies, along with some indicators of health such as the Infant Mortality Rates (IMR, death rate in the first year of life of all live births per 1000) and life expectancy at birth (World Health Organization, 1998).

In general these figures tend to show that poor countries (e.g. India, China, Ethiopia) have correspondingly poor indicators of health, with generally higher IMR and lower life expectancy at birth than in wealthier countries. This fits with other evidence (see Chapter 7) that socio-economic factors are a major influence on health. It is worth noting, however, that these relationships are not absolutely direct or linear. For example, above a certain level of GNP (e.g. comparing Spain and the Netherlands) health indicators are generally similar even for quite large differences in GNP. On the other hand, at the lower level of GNP a relatively small absolute difference in GNP (compare India and

Table 8.1 International comparisons

Country	GNP (US$)	IMR/1000	Life expectancy at birth (years)
Sweden	23,750	5	79
India	340	73	62
Spain	13,580	7	78
China	620	38	70
United Kingdom	18,700	6	77
Ethiopia	100	109	50
Netherlands	24,000	6	78
Japan	39,640	4	80
USA	26,980	7	77
Israel	15,920	7	78
New Zealand	14,340	7	77
Mexico	3320	31	72

Source: World Health Organization (1998).

Ethiopia) may signal the difference between severe poverty and absolute destitution with a corresponding large difference in health indicators (see also Chapter 14).

Control of economic influences on health

Economic factors can influence health in many ways, such as the impact of nutrition, housing, and water supplies. Governments can influence economic factors negatively through taxation of certain commodities and positively through subsidies on other commodities.

Taxation can be used to increase the price of goods and services, making them more expensive to buy. In this way, governments can reduce demand. Thus, adding (extra) tax to alcohol and tobacco makes these products more expensive, and fewer people will buy these products or they will buy less. A decrease in consumption of alcohol and tobacco at population level can be seen as an improvement in health behaviour, and will lead to health improvements in society. Governments can also use subsidies or tax reduction as policy instruments to make goods and services cheaper. This has led to an increase in cars which run on unleaded petrol, which in turn has lead to a slightly better environment and thus to fewer health problems.

Economic influences through spending on health care

We have seen that there are many different ways in which economic factors can affect health, most of which have little directly to do with health care provision. The figures given in Table 8.2 show spending on health services along with details of measures of health in different European countries. The expenditure figure includes both private and public health care costs to reflect total health care expenditure in countries with different types of health care systems.

Table 8.2 suggests that health care expenditure per head of the population has very little direct impact on two of the indicators of the state of a nation's health, namely infant mortality rates (IMR) and life expectancy. Countries with the highest expenditure per head of the population, such as Italy, spent nearly twice as much as, for example, Switzerland, yet they have the same IMR, and

Table 8.2 European comparisons

Country	1990 Health care expenditure *per capita* (US$)	IMR	Life expectancy for men at 40 (years)
Austria	1711	8.4	32.5
Belgium	1449	7.5	32.0
Denmark	1588	6.3	33.9
Finland	2046	7.8	31.8
France	1869	9.4	33.2
Germany	1511	8.7	32.9
Greece	359	5.4	36.4
Ireland	876	7.2	32.0
Italy	4655	7.5	33.7
Netherlands	1501	8.0	34.7
Portugal	383	7.0	32.0
Spain	831	6.6	34.5
Sweden	2343	8.8	34.9
Switzerland	2520	7.5	35.1
United kingdom	1039	6.1	32.7

Source: Murray & Lopez, World Health Organization (1994).

Switzerland actually has a higher life expectancy at 40 for men. This factor reflects a wide range of other influences on health (social cultures, etc.), as well as differences in the cost and efficiency of health care provision.

Regional differences in spending and health

There are such differences in both expenditure and the indicators of health between European countries, but also within a country as illustrated in Table 8.3. For example, within Scotland, government health care spending per person is almost 10% less in Lanarkshire than in other regions of Scotland. There are quite considerable variations in perinatal mortality rates (PNMR) and standardized death rates. As in Table 8.2 the regions with the lowest spending on health care do not necessarily have the highest PNMR and standardized death rates.

Political influence of legislation

Legislation in a number of areas can have an influence of health. Health can be improved or protected through legislation covering the workplace, the home, transport and travel, food and hygiene, water, and the environment. Legislation can come from different levels. For example, the European Directive on a maximum working week of 48 h has an impact on health, so has the British Government legislation on health and safety at work, and local council regulations on fire safety exists in public places. This protection can have a direct effect on health, as well as an indirect one. Legislation covering water quality

Table 8.3 Regional comparisons

Health board region	Spending per person (£)	Perinatal mortality rate	Death rate per 1000 (age/sex standardized)
Grampian	904	6.8	10.2
Tayside	937	7.5	10.9
Lothian	923	6.7	11.3
Greater Glasgow	890	7.7	13.0
Lanarkshire	858	10.1	12.7
Western Isles	955	6.5	11.8
Scotland	890	7.8	11.6

Source: ISD Scotland, 2000.

has an obvious direct impact, while legislation covering the dumping of rubbish can also have an indirect impact on our drinking water quality.

Political influence of social policy

Social policies are aimed at improving or protecting the general social well-being of individuals and communities. These policies are often aimed at the less privileged in society, such as the elderly, children, or the unemployed. Income support and benefits to those on low incomes are forms of social policy by governments, which will improve health and well-being. Pensions, social security, and child benefit are examples of assistance to targeted groups at risk in the community. Education is an important factor that influences health. Those with higher levels of education tend to be healthier than those of similar income who are less well educated.

Housing policy is another important example that affects particularly the health of people who live in council and rented accommodation. Poor, damp housing is associated with increased levels of respiratory diseases, such as asthma and ear infection. Housing standards control the basic tolerable living standards in terms of heating, lighting, access, water supply, and sanitation. There is good evidence that people who own their own homes tend to be healthier than people who live in council or privately rented accommodation, irrespective of income level. This may be partly explained by socio-demographic class differences (see Chapter 7), but it is also related to the level of control over the standard of the accommodation.

SUMMARY POINTS

- Many of the factors that influence health operate at the level of society and are, to an extent, out of the control of individuals.
- Study of economics helps explain the influences on distribution of resources of health care, whilst study of politics helps explain how governments can influence health care through policies, legislation, information, and education (as well as through economic control).
- Countries vary widely in the health of their populations, and that is related largely to economic and political factors.
- Within countries there can be regional differences that are due to a similar range of factors.
- Social policy, including education, employment, housing, and public health measures, has a much greater effect on the health of populations than has provision of medical services.

References and further reading

Acheson, D. (1998). *Independent Inquiry into Inequalities and Health*, Library 362.1 Ach. HMSO, London.

Detels, R. (1997). *Determinants of Health and Disease*, Oxford Textbook of Public Health, Vol. 1, 3rd edn. Oxford University Press, Oxford.

ISD Scotland (2000). *Scottish Health Statistics 1999*. Information and Statistics Division, National Health Service in Scotland, Edinburgh.

Marmot, M. & Wilkinson, K. (1999). *Social Determinanants of Health*. Oxford University Press, Oxford.

Murray, C.J.L. & Lopez, A.D. (1994). *Global Comparative Assessment in the Health Sector*. World Health Organization, Geneva.

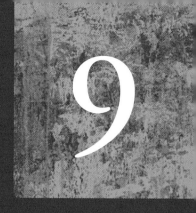

CHAPTER 9
Environmental influences on health

Environmental influences on health

The first things many people would think of when they hear the words 'environment and health' are probably pollution and Greenpeace. Environment, however, is wider than simply the physical environment. This is highlighted in the first part of this chapter that describes the basic constituents of the environment. It also highlights the major routes of exposure, the concept of exposure and dose, and it explains the differences between the concepts of hazard and risk. The second part uses classic examples to illustrate the impact of the environment on health. The third part describes the role of departments of Environmental and Consumer Protection.

Classification of the environment

The environment may be classified in a number of ways. The most frequently used classification sub-divides the environment into four components (Table 9.1), any, or all, or a combination of which may influence health status. When considering the possible environmental contribution to a patient's illness it may be helpful to consider each of these components in turn.

What constitutes a pollutant?

A polluting substance may be a solid, semi-solid, liquid, gas or sub-molecular particle. A substance or effect (for example, noise) is normally classified a pollutant if it adversely alters the environment by changing the growth rate of a species (for example, through causing infertility), or by interfering with the food chain, is toxic, or interferes with a person's health, comfort, or well being.

Routes of exposure

All chemicals are toxic under certain conditions of exposure. Even oxygen, which makes up roughly 20% of the atmosphere and which is fundamental to life, is toxic to humans if they are exposed to it at higher than atmospheric levels. We are constantly exposed to chemicals through our need for a continuous

Table 9.1 Classification of the environment

Environmental component	Description and examples
Biological	Comprises all flora and fauna. Includes pathogenic parasites (e.g. schistosoma), viruses (e.g. enteroviruses), and bacteria (cholera, typhoid). Sewage sludge.
Physical	Geological, geographical, climatic and meteorological characteristics. Noise, vibration, motor vehicles and other means of transport.
Chemical	Chemicals: organics and inorganics, drugs, alcohol, dust.
Social	Lifestyle characteristics such as smoking, diet, alcohol, occupation.

supply of food, water, and air. Requirements for food vary according to energy expenditure and habit but, at rest, the requirements for air and water are remarkably constant at 10–20 m^3 and 1–2 l per day, respectively. There are three major routes by which we come into contact with chemicals: the air, water, and soil (Fig. 9.1). There are other exposure routes and they differ in importance according to individual circumstances. The most important additional routes include the occupational setting, the home and lifestyle characteristics.

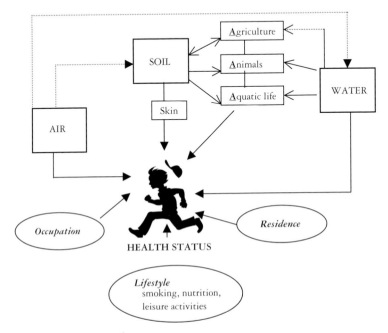

Fig. 9.1 The major routes of exposure.

Air

The majority of air pollutants are caused by industry or transport. The range of air pollutants is enormous, but the most common with regard to health include:

- particulate carbon matter and sulphur dioxide, which are by-products of power stations and the burning of fossil fuels;

- carbon dioxide and carbon monoxide that are by-products of power stations and motor vehicles, and a main contributor to the greenhouse effect;

- nitrogen oxides that are by-products of motor vehicles;

- heavy metals such as lead, cadmium, and nickel, which are by-products of burning petrol, the refining industry, and incineration.

The devastating fogs of last century, such as the London Fog 1952, the Meuse Valley Fog 1930, and the Pennsylvania Fog of 1948 were caused mainly by the burning of coal in domestic fires. The major pollutants they produced were particulate (carbon) matter and sulphur dioxide. With the introduction of smokeless zones and the burning of alternative fuels, these winter fogs have largely disappeared. Instead, we now have the summer smog of cities such as Los Angeles and Mexico City. Summer smog is caused by a build up of ozone, which is produced by the action of sunlight on volatile organic substances and nitrogen oxides. Motor vehicles are a major source of volatile organic substances and nitrogen oxides.

The belching chimneys of industrial Britain and Western Europe are less common, and more controlled than previously. However, industry still contributes significantly to the overall burden of air pollution. Many of the modern day pollutants are less visible; gaining knowledge about their impact on health and on the environment, either singly or, more importantly, as part of a cocktail of exposure, is the challenge facing scientists over the next 50 years.

Weather conditions can greatly exacerbate air borne pollution. Boisterous winds help to disperse air pollution, whereas high pressure weather systems can result in the trapping of air pollution at ground level.

High pressure system → *anticyclonic weather conditions* → *temperature inversion** → *trapping air pollutants at ground level*
*Temperature inversions are formed when a layer of warm air overlies and prevents cold air from rising.

A classic example of air pollution exacerbated by weather conditions was the London fogs of the 1950s. They are described in detail later in this chapter.

Soil

Soil may become polluted in a number of ways, for example from:

♦ industry, either as fall out from chimneys or as leachate from waste dumps (industrial or municipal);

♦ use of herbicides, pesticides, and fungicides in agriculture;

♦ the spreading of sewage sludge;

♦ the deposition of heavy metals from exhaust fumes of motor vehicles and industrial chimneys.

Pollution of the ground → contaminated crops/animals → contamination of the food chain → exposure of humans

A classic example of contaminated land resulting in ill health occurred at Love Canal, a landfill site near Niagara Falls, USA. The site had been used as a chemical and municipal waste disposal site from the 1930s until 1953. Homes were built next to the landfill. In the late 1960s there were complaints from residents about chemical odours in the home basements. By the early 1970s public concern had grown appreciably, and environmental and health investigations were undertaken. Although none of the reported studies have (so far) reported a causal link between the site and specific ill health, there is a high incidence of social and psychological morbidity in the vicinity. Even in the face of strong suggestive evidence, establishing a causal link indisputably is often impossible. In these cases, evidence is weighed differently by different parties.

Water

Water may be polluted either through run off from the land (which might be contaminated by pesticides or by fertilizers used in agriculture) or by the dumping of industrial waste into the rivers and sea.

Pollution of the water → contaminated vegetation → contaminated fish → contamination of the food chain → exposure of humans

A classic example of contaminated water adversely affecting health happened in Japan in 1953. A mysterious neurological disorder affected residents of Minamata Bay. The symptoms included polyneuritis, cerebellar ataxia, and cortical blindness. The suspected culprit was identified as contaminated fish from the bay. The symptoms were so similar to poisoning by mercury that the epidemiologists looked for a source of organic mercury. A factory was found to be dumping mercury into the bay.

Natural pollution

Not all pollution is caused by man. Nature contributes appreciable quantities. For example, the main source of exposure to radiation in the UK is from natural sources, such as radon gas from bedrock (for instance in Aberdeen and Cornwall), from buildings and from food. Fallout from volcanic eruptions causes airborne pollution, which can affect global weather patterns. Airborne pollen from plants causes respiratory and skin sensitivity in susceptible people.

Exposure and dose

Exposure should be measured both in terms of level and duration. Some pollutants act immediately in producing adverse health outcomes, such as in the London Fog episode. Others produce effects only after prolonged exposure. Most chemicals that accumulate in the body, such as lead and mercury, or hazards that have an accumulative affect, such as radiation or noise, require prolonged exposures to provoke adverse health outcomes. When trying to establish the relationship between exposure, and an environmental pollutant it is important to quantify as accurately as possible the level and duration of exposure needed to produce a health effect.

For many pollutants there is a number of effects ranging from subtle covert physiological or biochemical changes, to overt severe illness. The higher the dose, the more severe the effect. This relationship between dose and severity of health outcome is known as dose-effect or dose-response. Knowledge about the dose-effect relationship is important because it provides the foundation for the setting of safety standards.

Hazards and risk

The word hazard is derived from the Arabic word for gaming dice and describes the potential to cause harm. Risk is a measure of the likelihood of harm occurring from exposure to a hazard. How a person views a hazard is dependent upon their perception of the risk or the expected benefit to be derived from exposure to the hazard. For example, the hazard of smoking is generally well acknowledged by society; it causes lung cancer, bronchitis, emphysema, and heart disease, it contributes to many other illnesses and it reduces life expectancy. Yet, 34% of the British public continues to smoke. The hazard is appreciated, but the risk is not necessarily acknowledged—possibly because of the benefit (pleasure) derived, because of other competing needs (peer group pressure), or because of the ostrich effect (it won't happen to me).

Two people exposed to the same amount of a hazard will not necessarily experience the same degree of illness. Not everyone exposed to cigarette smoking

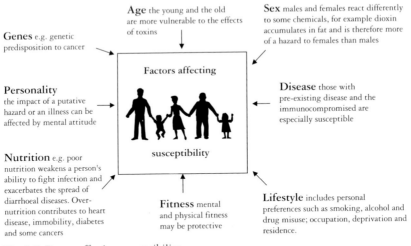

Age the young and the old are more vulnerable to the effects of toxins

Sex males and females react differently to some chemicals, for example dioxin accumulates in fat and is therefore more of a hazard to females than males

Genes e.g. genetic predisposition to cancer

Personality the impact of a putative hazard or an illness can be affected by mental attitude

Disease those with pre-existing disease and the immunocompromised are especially susceptible

Nutrition e.g. poor nutrition weakens a person's ability to fight infection and exacerbates the spread of diarrhoeal diseases. Over-nutrition contributes to heart disease, immobility, diabetes and some cancers

Factors affecting susceptibility

Fitness mental and physical fitness may be protective

Lifestyle includes personal preferences such as smoking, alcohol and drug misuse; occupation, deprivation and residence.

Fig. 9.2 Factors affecting susceptibility.

gets lung cancer, not everyone exposed to the cholera vibrio gets cholera and not everyone exposed to the flu virus gets flu. The risk to an individual from a hazard is determined also by that person's susceptibility. Susceptibility varies between individuals, and is the sum of a person's life experiences and genetic makeup (Fig. 9.2).

The Environment and Health

Whoever wishes to investigate medicine properly, should proceed thus: in the first place to consider the seasons of the year, and what effects each of them produces . . . Then the cold winds, the hot and the cold, especially such as are common to all countries, and then such as are peculiar to each locality. We must also consider the qualities. In the same manner, when one comes into a city to which he is a stranger, he ought to consider its situation how it lies to the winds and the rising of the sun; for its influence is not the same whether it lies to the north or to the south, to the rising or to the setting sun. These things one ought to consider most attentively, and concerning the waters which the inhabitants use, whether they be marshy and soft, or hard, and running from elevated and rocky situations, and then if saltish and unfit for cooking; and the ground, whether it be naked and deficient in water, or wooded and well watered, and whether it lies in a hollow, confined situation, or is elevated and cold: and the mode in which the inhabitants live, and what are their pursuits, whether they are fond of drinking and eating to excess, and given to indolence, or are fond of exercise and labour, and not given to excess eating and drinking. (Adams 1849)

The general idea that the environment can influence health has its origins in antiquity. There have been several classic studies demonstrating this relationship, but one of the earliest in Great Britain was the investigation of cholera epidemics by a London General Practitioner, John Snow.

The London Cholera epidemic 1848–54

Several water companies supplied London with water. In 1849 Snow observed that the cholera rates were particularly high in an area of London, which was supplied by two companies—the Lambeth Company, and the Southwark and Vauxhall Company. Both of these companies obtained their water supply from a location on the River Thames that was particularly polluted with sewage. Between 1849–54 the Lambeth Company relocated its collection point to a less polluted position in the River Thames. By 1854 the two companies were supplying roughly two-thirds of the London population living south of the river. In this area, the two companies had interweaved their water mains to such an extent that households in the same street were receiving water from either of the two sources.

The natural experiment

In 1854 another epidemic of cholera struck London. Snow counted the number of households supplied by each water company and calculated cholera death rates per 10,000 households, for the first 7 weeks of the epidemic. He then compared these rates to those for the remainder of London. The results were unequivocal. The mortality rates from cholera in households supplied by the Southwark & Vauxhall Company were 8–9 times higher than in households supplied by the Lambeth company (Table 9.2).

Snow's conclusions

These findings, together with another investigation of the so-called Broad Street Pump outbreak, led Snow to put forward the theory of a 'cholera poison', which was transmittable by water. Thirty years later, the cholera vibrio was identified.

Table 9.2 Mortality rates for cholera, London, 1854

Water source	Number of households	Deaths from cholera	Rate per 10,000
Southwark & Vauxhall	40,046	1263	315
Lambeth	26,107	98	38
Remainder of London	256,423	1422	56

Another classic example that demonstrates the impact of the environment on health is the London Fog episode of 1952.

London Fog

A dense fog covered the Greater London area during 5–8 December 1952. During this time there was a sudden and enormous rise in mortality, which far exceeded anything previously recorded in a similar period of fog. The number of deaths in excess of those expected for the first 3 weeks of December was between 3500 and 4000 (Fig. 9.3). The population of Greater London at this time was roughly 8 million.

The fog was particularly dense and did not lift at all during 5–8 December. It led to an accumulation of pollutants in the fog, to which the waste products of the burning of domestic coal (i.e. particulate matter and sulphur dioxide) contributed significantly (Fig. 9.4).

Analysis of the death certificates showed that the increase in deaths was in the *susceptible* population of the old, young, and ill (particularly those with chronic respiratory or cardiac disease). Between 60 and 70% of the deaths were in people over 60 years, and the death rate was doubled in children under one year.

This fog episode instigated the Clean Air Act 1956. A major influence of this act was a restriction in the burning of domestic coal fires.

The impact of the environment on health has been appreciated since antiquity, but it has taken the more recent major disasters to draw public and political attention to the potential hazards contained in the environment.

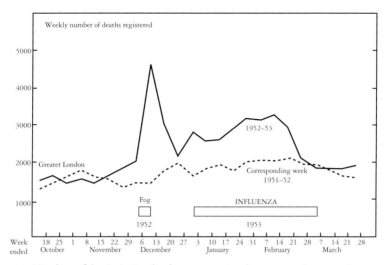

Fig. 9.3 Numbers of deaths in London between 18 October 1952 and 28 March 1953 compared with the corresponding dates in 1951–52.

Source: Ministry of Health, 1954.

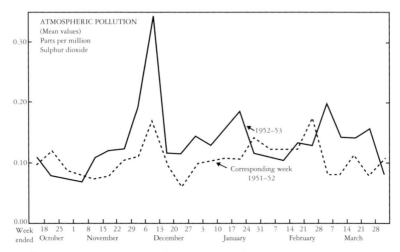

Fig. 9.4 Sulphur dioxide in London between 18 October 1952 and 28 March 1953 compared with the corresponding dates in 1951–52.

Source: Ministry of Health, 1954.

A brief synopsis of three major environmental disasters

ICMESA Chemical Plant, Seveso, Northern Italy

In 1976 in Seveso, a chemical reactor exploded at a factory that made trichlorophenol. A toxic cloud formed, which was heavily contaminated with dioxin. Short-term health outcomes included an increase in the spontaneous abortion rate and a high incidence of chloracne (an unpleasant skin condition). Long-term health outcomes are still uncertain, but the incidence of several cancers and cardiovascular risk appear to be raised. Epidemiological monitoring was instigated at the time of the accident and is still continuing. Studies on workers in industries that manufacture trichlorophenol show only an increased incidence of chloracne; no other cause of death is consistently raised.

Union Carbide Factory, Bhopal, India

In 1984 in Bhopal, approximately 40 tonnes of highly toxic methyl isocyanate (MIC) gas escaped into the atmosphere. Roughly one-quarter of the town's inhabitants were thought to be exposed to the highly toxic aerosol: 2500 people died immediately and as many as 250,000 were injured, many seriously, many permanently. Long-term health consequences so far identified are permanent respiratory and neurological damage (blindness). There was a high loss of life for at least three reasons. First, the close proximity of the workers' shanty homes to the factory (around the perimeter fence in many instances). MIC is heavier than air and most of the shanty homes were single story ramshackle shacks. Secondly, the explosion happened at 01.00 h when many were asleep. Thirdly, there is some evidence that, in underdeveloped countries, some industries practise without the same level of care as would be expected in developed countries. The World Health Organization reports that there are no effective legal requirements to deal with pollution in the workplace and surrounding areas in many developing countries.

Nuclear reactor, Chernobyl, Russia

In 1986, a nuclear reactor exploded in Chernobyl. According to the available reports 825,000 people were contaminated. A toxic cloud formed over Chernobyl and following a change in wind direction, a cloud trail of 2000 km containing Caesium 137 was detected in 20 countries. Thirty deaths and 300 severe cases of radiation burning occurred immediately in personnel working in the plant and in those fighting the fires around Chernobyl. The long-term health consequences to the exposed populations are very difficult to quantify. It has been estimated that radiation measuring about one million curies was released at the time of the accident into the Russian environment. It is suggested that if one million people were exposed and each received 1 rem of radiation then only 100–200 additional fatal cancers would occur in that population. It has also been estimated that for most exposed populations individual doses range from a fraction of a year's background radiation to between 2 and 4 years'. Thus, for an individual, there is only a minute risk of a serious health effect. It is likely that we shall never know the true incidence of cancer caused by the accident as the epidemiological tools do not exist to distinguish these cancers from the 190,000 spontaneous cancers that would ordinarily occur in that population.

Conclusions

The potential environmental influences on health are many and they will continue to expand, as society becomes more and more complex. Responsibility for protecting the environment rests with us all, but in matters to do with a person's health special responsibility falls to doctors—particularly public health specialists and general practitioners—and to environmental health officers. Environmental health officers are based in local or regional departments of Environmental and Consumer Protection throughout the UK. They provide many services and functions, and ultimately exist to protect the health of the public. For example, they co-ordinate refuse collection, street cleaning, special and clinical waste collection, recycling, pest, and animal control. They are the enforcement authority for food safety, health and safety, noise and pollution control, public health nuisances, port health, consumer safety, fair trading, and weights and measures. General Practitioners and Public Health Medicine

Specialists with responsibility for communicable disease work closely with departments of Environmental and Consumer Protection for a variety of reasons, but in particular during outbreaks of gastrointestinal diseases.

SUMMARY POINTS

- The environment is usefully classified as Biological (all flora and fauna), Physical (e.g. geology, weather, noise, and vibration), Chemical (organic and inorganic matter), and Social (smoking, diet, occupation): a classification that emphasizes that the environment is not purely physical.

- All chemicals (even, e.g. oxygen) are potentially toxic and may pollute through air, water, and soil, or through the house and work. Important air pollutants include sulphur and carbon dioxides, nitrogen oxides, and traces of heavy metals. Soil contaminants include herbicides and pesticides and water pollution, similarly, includes pesticides and fertilizers. Other natural hazards include radiation and volcanic eruptions.

- Some pollutants have immediate effects, but many take a longer time to accumulate in the body and cause harm.

- Risk is a measure of the likelihood of harm occurring from exposure to a hazard, such as a pollutant. Different individuals may be more or less impervious to a hazard, depending on genetic make-up and other factors.

- The chapter describes the classic examples of the London cholera epidemic, 1848; the London Fog of 1952 and three other major industrial disasters; and ends with a brief description of environmental and public health organization in the United Kingdom.

References and further reading

Adams, F. (1849). *The Genuine Works of Hippocrates on Airs, Waters, and Places*, Vol. I, p. 190. The Sydenham Society, London.

British Medical Association (1998). *Health and Environmental Impact Assessment: an integrated approach*. Earthscan Publications Ltd, London.

Cassens, B.J. (1992). *Preventive Medicine and Public Health*, 2nd edn. Williams & Wilkins, Baltimore.

Last, J.M. (1987). *Public Health and Human Ecology*. Appleton & Large, New York.

Ministry of Health (1954). *Mortality and Morbidity During the London Fog of December 1952*. A report by a Committee of Departmental Officers and Expert Advisers appointed by the Minister of Health. HMSO, London.

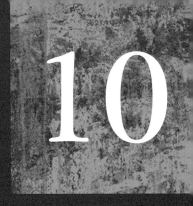

10

CHAPTER 10

Influence of mental processes on health

Influence of mental processes on health

Introduction

There is enormous variation between individuals in the nature of their mental processes. The psychological environment affects all areas of health, as well as being an important aspect of health itself. The challenge in the community is to identify (if they exist) boundaries between a healthy mental life, and what happens when the signs and symptoms of mental disorder appear. This chapter summarizes approaches to understanding the mental processes that contribute to:

- Sensation, perception, and consciousness
- Cognition
- Learning and memory
- Language and communication
- Intelligence
- Emotions
- Personality

Sensation, perception, and consciousness

Perception is more than the simple acts of seeing or hearing. These are sensations. When a stimulus is perceived, its properties are acted upon by the mind. The brain brings experience of similar earlier perceptions to bear on this active process. Sensation, in contrast, is a passive process. The fact that perception is active means that the perceptual process can be tricked by certain types of stimuli, especially if these are ambiguous. Figure 10.1 shows an optical illusion of this type in which the subject may be seen either as a young or as an old woman. In healthy mental life, illusions most commonly arise when attention cannot be properly focused or there are competing, similar sensations of uncertain significance. This manner of experience can occur on falling asleep (hypnogogic) or on waking (hypnopompic). In these normal states of mind,

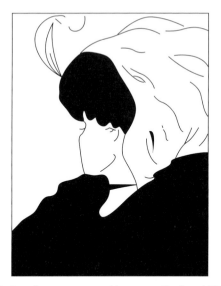

Fig. 10.1 Optical illusion of a young or an old woman. (Boring, 1930).

consciousness is said to be lowered. A hallucination is the perception of an external stimulus in the absence of any appropriate stimulus. Perceptual abnormalities like hallucinations and illusions occur commonly in severe types of mental illness. However, the boundary between 'healthy' and 'unhealthy' perceptual abnormalities is indistinct.

Mental space and altered consciousness

The term consciousness implies awareness of experience. Practical definitions of consciousness rely on observation of those phenomena believed to depend crucially on the presence of consciousness. Thus, consciousness may be detected by behaviour that shows that an individual can differentiate between external stimuli, and between internal feelings and the external world. This behaviour relies on the ability to shift attention at will. This kind of differentiation is observed in discriminatory behaviour that can be elicited during mental examination. The conscious individual is aware and, in being aware, is also knowing (cognitive). This individual can distinguish what is known from that which is as yet undifferentiated in the experienced world. A conscious individual is capable of self-reflection. When we speak or write about consciousness we visualize a space in which mental images can be displayed. We talk about ideas being at 'the front' or 'the back of our minds', or we may have 'deep' or 'open minds'. We can even consider ideas from the 'corners of our minds'. Popular terms for different states of consciousness include unconscious and subconscious. These are sometimes used synonymously, but do not mean the same thing. Sigmund Freud introduced the term 'unconscious' to denote ideas that could easily be brought to mind (see emotions below). Other states of consciousness include sleep, dreaming, and hypnosis. Drugs may bring about alternative states of consciousness.

Cognition

Psychologists use the term cognition to describe thinking processes. Classical notions of logical thinking are best illustrated by mathematical rules, where correct application of the rules (addition, division, multiplication, or subtraction) will invariably produce the one and only correct answer. Some, but not many, human problems may be susceptible to this kind of thinking. Most human thinking, however, involves judgement, assessment of risk, weighing up evidence, and deciding which is the best of a number of posssible choices or solutions. A common example is given in Box 1. The process described there, by which lay people decide which action to take about symptoms of illness, is probably not greatly different from the general way that doctors diagnose illness.

BOX 1 How do you deal with a headache?

Most of us get headaches from time to time. Think back to the last time you had a headache (or some similar common symptom). We expect that, like most lay people, you were able to do some simple clinical problem solving, in order to decide what best to do. For example, the headache might have followed a pattern that you recognize from previous experience, e.g. like a 'hangover' from the party the night before, like a migraine if you are a known migraine sufferer, or like the sort of tension headache you have following a late night studying for exams. However, the headache might also have been a 'new' type for you. How do you decide what to do, in particular, whether or not you need medical advice? In general, this process is one of weighing up evidence for and against the likelihood or probability, of a particular possibility, like meningitis, as against others, such as a simpler kind of illness, like a common cold. Of course, common colds or 'flu like illnesses are, by definition, much more common than meningitis and, therefore, much more likely to be the answer. Thus, in this process there is also an assessment of the degree of risk attached to each possibility. Obviously, much more weight needs to be given to the serious possibilities like meningitis, so that 'to be on the safe side' most people would seek medical advice if they could not be sure of the cause and thought that a more serious cause was possible, even though unlikely. Much of the time, however, people are able to self-treat or manage common symptoms, like headaches, by applying this kind of thinking, which uses analogies with previous experience, strategies and rules of thumb. This kind of thinking is sometimes described as 'heuristic', as opposed to the rule bound, stepwise 'algorithms', characterized by mathematical logic. The aim is to select the solution that is the most likely to be successful, judging the likelihood and the risks from amongst other possible solutions.

Learning and memory

Information acquired during learning is stored in memory. Learning experiments examine behavioural changes over time in response to the same repeated stimulus. For convenience, learning is studied in animals and memory is studied in humans. Historical studies of learning began with 'conditioning' experiments where novel relationships between a stimulus and response were induced by association. Ivan Pavlov taught dogs to associate the presentation of food with the sound of a bell. Usually, dogs salivate when food is presented. After 'conditioning', salivation can be induced by the sound of a bell alone (classical conditioning). Another form of learning used in animal experiments is termed 'operant conditioning'. The animal (the 'operant') learns to associate a reward with a behaviour previously unrelated to rewards of any kind. In both types of learning, the link may be extinguished by persistent absence of any reward (food in 'classical conditioning' and 'operant conditioning'). Likewise, learning is reinforced by repeated rewards.

Memory is of several different types. In human experiments, the duration of retention of memory forms the simplest decision. 'Iconic memory' is placed in a store lasting about half a second before transfer (if required) into short-term memory lasting about 15 seconds. Long-term memory requires information to be sorted and encoded before being placed in stores from where it can be retrieved. Amnesia (or failure to retrieve memories) can be caused by a failure to encode or retrieve. In one view of the mind, there are arrays of memory banks ready to recognize sensations and contribute to active perceptual processing of this information. The memory banks also have the capacity to reflect on memories as they are retrieved ('thoughts about thoughts'). The memory banks are arranged so that they can process shared types of information. Everyday life is available in terms of a specific context (such as 'what is in the timetable this morning?'). This is known as 'episodic memory'. More general knowledge is stored in 'semantic memory' and answers factual questions, such as 'who won the football world cup in 1970?' Episodic and semantic memory are available for conscious access and can be brought to mind. Other types of memory are certainly not available in this way. These include motor skills like a perfect golf swing, or other automatic and unconscious behaviours.

Language and communication

Social behaviours in organized groups of animals rely on some form of communication. Although humans have the only well-understood form of language, other animals, particularly birds, probably have complex forms of language.

When language is used effectively, other properties of the spoken word (e.g. pitch and intonation) convey a substantial part of the meaning. 'Non-verbal communications' like facial expression, eye movements, and body posture also help convey meaning. Helpful and effective communication in medicine takes account of the use of language in ways that combine the elements of the spoken word, and appropriate non-verbal signals to convey genuineness, warmth, encouragement, and empathy. These skills can be used consciously in a responsible and responsive way to indicate sensitivity to the emotional issues raised, to establish trust, and to sustain a helpful, therapeutic relationship. The converse is also true—clashes in communication may be needlessly provoked when too little attention is paid to the necessary establishment of the essential components of communication. Sometimes, something as simple as giving advice can become fraught with difficulty because the client/patient presents spoken and non-verbal communications that are at odds with one another; for example, smiling when describing distress.

Intelligence

Intelligence is difficult to define and can only be measured by proxy. The preceding descriptions of mental health in life have emphasized similarities between individuals. The phenomenon of intelligence represents a special view on many aspects of thinking and memory that is informed by these descriptions, but which should be carefully distinguished from them. For example, intelligence tests measure performance on set tasks that require mental ability to solve correctly. Human performance, in turn, is influenced by factors as diverse as motivation, the perceived purpose of the test, emotional feelings perhaps unrelated to the test, familiarity with test materials or sessions, hunger, thirst; the list is very long. Ideally, intelligence test results should inform about the optimum capacity of the individual to do those things that require intelligence to complete (eliminating these other factors as far as possible).

Intelligence tests are designed to compare individuals. They do not give absolute values of mental ability. Most intelligence tests contain items to evaluate ability with vocabulary, arithmetic, puzzle solving, spatial reasoning and sentence comprehension. The convention in childhood and adolescence is to compare intelligence test scores between children at different ages using the intelligence quotient:

$$IQ = Mental\ age \times 100/Chronological\ age$$

Not surprisingly, unless test conditions are carefully regulated, IQ test scores can vary widely in the same person over time. These and related observations have suggested to some that IQ is not a useful concept and can be discarded. Recent studies, however, indicate that there remains much research value in studies of IQ (e.g. in molecular genetics). However, other data on the sources of individual differences are probably of more interest in, for example, job selection or planning the education of a child.

The measurement of intelligence has generated theories on the nature or structure of intelligence. Theorists differ in their interpretation of the relationships between scores on different types of mental ability test (e.g. verbal reasoning versus spatial ability). Some believe that there is an underlying general ability that contributes importantly to all special types of mental ability; others argue that these abilities are independent. These types of study examine what is known as the 'psychometric model'. Current theories seek to link these ideas to recent advances in molecular genetics and the neuroscience of information processing.

Emotions

Emotions are subjective feeling states experienced by individuals, but not observable by others, although associated physical manifestations may 'give away' the emotion to an observer.

Sigmund Freud studied the origins of *anxiety*. He was very much influenced by prevailing late nineteenth century ideas about the nature and sources of mental energy, which he thought could be diverted or repressed, but never destroyed. His first ideas concerned the nature of instinctual drives (food, thirst, sex, and self-preservation) among which he gave primacy to sex drive. He divided mental life into two domains, conscious and unconscious. Within the unconscious domain, he firmly placed a primitive instinctual drive (the 'id') towards pleasurable rewards, but modified or checked by the 'super-ego' representing acquired attitudes, values, and moral character. When the two conflicted unconscious anxiety would be generated and in order to maintain 'ego integrity', the ego could employ certain 'defence mechanisms' (Table 10.1). Freud believed that unconscious conflict of this form was the origin of anxiety, which accompanied many types of minor mental illness termed 'neurosis'. Freud also found similarities

Table 10.1 Some common mental defence mechanisms

Defence Mechanism	Example
Denial	Pretend the facts are wrong when faced by the truth
Repression	'I don't know that, I never did'
Isolation	'I know what you're saying, but it's of no importance'
Sublimation	'I'll just go and have a good game of squash'
Displacement	'What do you mean I'm angry! I'm not, it's you that's treating me badly. You're fed up with me as a patient'
Projection	'I'm not bothered at all, I wouldn't be here if my wife wasn't so upset'!
Reaction formation	'Of course I'm not bothered about it, in fact I've never been less worried'
Regression	'I can't do anything, I can't take part in any decision. Just let the doctor decide'

between the experience of grief in bereavement and depressive disorders: in depression, the loss was not real from the outside world, but occurred in the internal mental world. This led John Bowlby to suggest the 'attachment theory' of the emotions. Attachments are bonds between individuals that are lasting and provide us with sources of support when faced by adversity. Attachments develop first within families and then extend to friendships at school or workplace. Breaking such attachments in childhood leads to 'separation anxiety'. Emotional maturity involves using 'coping strategies' to solve gradually more complex social problems. Erik Erikson summarized these problems, their solutions and the consequences of failure as 'crises'.

The first crisis occurs in the first year of life as the problem of trust (basic trust versus mistrust). How safe is it to extend the trust of your mother to trusting others including strangers? The next crisis, between ages 1 and 3, concerns the first ventures outside the safety of the family (autonomy versus shame and doubt). The third, between ages 3 and 6, describes the problem of further development of activities outside the family with friends, and addresses the question of taking the initiative in these matters or remaining distant and developing a sense of guilt that one is not doing so (initiative versus guilt). At school, success derives from application of hard work, contributions to group activities, and securing the praise and approval of teachers. This crisis is termed 'industry versus inferiority'. In adolescence, facing separation from parents and the establishment of a personal identity with responsibilities for one's decisions, future, friends, and so on, is the basis of emotional life in adulthood. This crisis is termed 'identity versus role confusion'.

Personality

One view of personal development from childhood to adolescence is of a 'developmental' approach to the study of personality. Other approaches derive from the view that underlying all various types of personality there are several major classes, to one of which an individual may approximate. The third approach to understanding personality is the idea that personality has a fundamental structure, a bit like the steel frame of a modern concrete piece of 'slab architecture'. The design of this framework is consistent from one personality structure to another—variability occurs in the strength, shape, and size of individual pieces. This is the 'dimensional' approach to personality.

Definition: personality is used to describe the constellation of attitudes, temperament, and character that most satisfactorily distinguishes people as unique individuals. These characteristics are present from late childhood, are relatively enduring traits, and are distinct from symptoms such as depression or emotional states that are transient.

In some studies of large numbers of individuals, certain personality traits have been found to be associated with ill health. The best known of these is the association of 'Type A' behaviour with increased risk of coronary artery disease. This is more fully described in Chapter 17. In brief, Type A behaviour is characterized by high competitiveness, need to achieve, aggression, impatience, restlessness, hyper-alertness, and sensitivity to time pressure. Type B behaviour is the converse of these traits. However, although this typification is probably the best attempt to link personality factors to illness, it is still generally acknowledged that it works better at an epidemiological (population) level than on a particular individual, because any such classification can only be crude, given the uniqueness of individual personalities.

If personality is really unique then no classification of categories or measurement of dimensions will provide an adequate solution. In these circumstances, an 'idiothetic' approach is essential. This is preferred by many psychotherapists. The reasoning is simple. If we accept that one of the main tasks of personality theory is to make accurate predictions of an individual's behaviour in quite specific future circumstances then it might follow that the more information we had about an individual (especially their behaviour in response to similar past circumstances) the more accurate would be our prediction. This is termed the 'prospective validity' of a personality measure. It is what some occupational psychologists try to achieve when matching individuals with jobs on the basis of pencil and paper personality tests. So far, no method of personality measurement has met the 'gold standard' set by predictive validity.

The 'normothetic' approach' is based on the recognition of differences between an individual and a sample believed to be representative of the population at large. These differences are measured on scales devised to detect similarities between large groups, while at the same time identifying individuals who are obvious 'outliers'. These scales are used in psychometrics where they contribute to personality questionnaires. The results of these questionnaires can be analysed so that they emphasize similarities between individuals and estimate how alike a single individual might be to a typical category of personality. Alternatively, the questionnaire data may be analysed so that similarities between items of the test (not individuals) are detected. This is the basis of the dimensional approach to personality popularized by Hans Eysenck.

Apart from these formal systems of personality measurement, specialist practitioners in the field of mental health may explicitly assess individual personality during the clinical interview by, for example, exploring the individual's use of defence mechanisms (Table 10.1) and their adherence to society's standard of 'normal' behaviour.

However, a basic understanding of theories of personality will help all health professionals to understand individual patients, their illnesses (whether these are predominantly psychological and physical), and their reaction to illness.

Finally, this chapter has dealt with 'normal' variations in personality. In Chapter 17 we deal more with disorders in personality and how these affect behaviour, health, and vulnerability to disapproval by society in general.

SUMMARY POINTS

- ◆ The mental processes are an important basis of health and influence all aspects of health.
- ◆ The boundaries between a healthy mental life and a mental disorder may be difficult or impossible to define.
- ◆ This chapter summarizes the main conventional approaches to understanding the mental processes that contribute to sensation, perception, and consciousness; cognition; learning and memory; language and communication; intelligence; and emotions.

References and further reading

Boring, E. G. (1930). A new ambiguous figure. *American Journal of Psychology*, 42, 444–5.

Porter, M., Alder, B. & Abraham, C. (1999). *Psychology and Sociology Applied to Medicine: an illustrated colour text*. Churchill Livingston, Edinburgh.

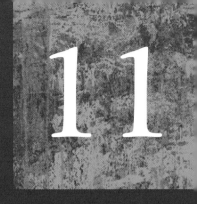

CHAPTER 11
Influence of age on health

CHAPTER 11
Influence of age on health

Introduction

Age has an important influence on all dimensions of health, and affects the aetiology, impact, and management of most illnesses. This chapter will examine associations between age and health throughout the life span, and introduce ideas about the interplay between age-changes, environment, lifestyle, and disease. It will also explain attitudes to age that can have an influence on health and disease. It will address the issues of advocacy and ageism, and discuss how paternalistic attitudes affect children and how ageist attitudes may affect the health of older people.

General background

The two specialties of medicine that are defined primarily in terms of the patient's age are Child Health (Paediatrics) and Medicine for the Elderly (Geriatric Medicine). Some researchers use the word 'ageing' to cover the whole of this period, but we will adopt the more usual convention of 'growth and development' to cover the period from conception to young adulthood and 'ageing' to cover the period from middle age onwards. The exact points at which these processes begin and end depend on the medical and social context, and are also subject to individual variation.

At the extremes of life, age tends to be a matter of pride. The child of $4\frac{3}{4}$ is proud that he or she has progressed from the relative immaturity of being $4\frac{1}{2}$, while the 90-year-old on a television game show gets a round of applause simply on the basis of this chronological fact. However, much more ambivalent attitudes are often found in the middle-aged. At the beginning of life, change is particularly rapid, but is usually associated with a keen sense of anticipation, and an over-riding confidence in the future and the new phase of life about to be entered. It is much less common for the transition from adulthood to old age to be viewed in such a positive light, but older people who are financially secure and medically fit sometimes regard old age as the best time of their lives. We should avoid stereotyping at any age, but the risk is particularly high in older people as they often have very stereotyped ideas of themselves.

Similarities between the very young and the very old: the role of homeostasis

Homeostasis is defined as 'a tendency to stability in the normal body status (internal environment) of the organism'. Homeostatic reserve tends to increase during development, reach a plateau in adult life, and decline thereafter. Indeed, one of the definitions of ageing is a progressive loss of adaptability as time passes. As we grow older, we become less able to react adaptively to challenges from the external or internal environment (Evans & Williams 1992). Because of impaired homeostasis, very young and very old individuals may be overwhelmed by stressful situations that would lead to more minor problems in younger adults.

Some examples of similarities between the very young and the very old, which probably arise from impaired ability to counter physical stresses and/or disease are:

♦ Respiratory disease, which has its major impact at either end of the life span, being the single commonest cause for hospital admission under the age of 5 and a major reason for hospital admission in old age.

♦ Acute delirium as the result of infection and fever, which is commonest in childhood and old age.

Survival rates after trauma and burns tend to follow a U-shaped curve with the highest mortality rates in the very young and very old.

Figure 11.1 is a stylized diagram of lung function (corrected for body size), age, respiratory disease, and smoking based on a cross-sectional survey carried out on people of different ages. The patterns shown in Fig. 11.1 appear deceptively

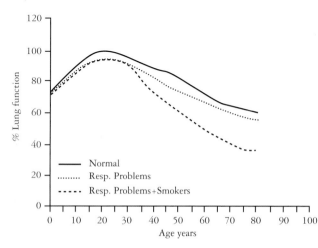

Fig. 11.1 The interaction of development, ageing, environment, lifestyle, and disease.

simple. In 'normal' people, lung function appears to increase until about the age of 20, to remain stable for about 15 years after that, and then gradually to decline. (Incidentally, this general pattern is also seen in cross-sectional studies of many other body systems, including cardiac function and renal function). Patients with respiratory diseases have lung function values that follow the same general pattern, but average values are lower. After the age of 40, smokers have a much more rapid decline in lung function than non-smokers.

BOX 1

Looking at Fig. 11.1, how many of the following statements are true?

1. The main period of lung growth is between birth and 10 years of age.

2. It is normal and inevitable that you will lose lung function after the age of 35.

3. Information such as that given in Fig. 11.1 is useful in interpreting the clinical importance of a lung function test in an *individual* patient who you have just met for the first time, and who has not previously had a lung function test.

4. It is safe to smoke until you are 40 and it is not worth giving up smoking once you are 70.

5. It is useful to think in terms of three separate processes affecting function:

   (i) normal development and ageing;
   (ii) environment and lifestyle;
   (iii) disease.

For the moment, jot down a few quick responses to these five statements. Return to them at the end of the chapter and see if your answers has changed.

Early influences: normal development, health, and disease

Normality or abnormality?

In the field of Child Health the inter-relationship of normality and disease is complex. In the fetus, neonate, and child, anatomical and physiological changes occur at a very rapid rate. One of the great achievements of Child Health is that a great deal of data are now available about 'normal' values for various functions at various stages of development. The interpretation of such data, along with the decision whether or not to intervene when apparent abnormalities are present, are two of the central skills needed by the specialist in Child Health.

Effects of early negative and positive influences on lifelong health

'The child is the father of the man'. This famous quotation by William Wordsworth refers to emotional and social development, but recent evidence suggests that, in addition to these factors, very important physical effects of early growth and development are present in the infant and young child and even in the fetus. Recent evidence, suggests that the intra-uterine environment may have lifelong consequences for adult health (Barker 1992). This is not surprising, considering the complex organ development that takes place from the fertilized ovum to the infant at term and the huge amount of physical growth that occurs during intra-uterine life. Peak velocity of growth occurs at about 18–20 weeks of gestational age, and at no time during subsequent growth and development is this rate of growth exceeded. However, this fetal programming hypothesis has been challenged as environmental influences may operate throughout the whole of life (see review by Kramer & Joseph 1996).

Figure 11.2 based on data collected by Barker *et al.* (1991), shows the relationship of birth weight in pounds to standardized mortality ratio for chronic obstructive lung disease and carcinoma of the lung. Whereas the mortality from lung cancer is not much influenced by birth weight, mortality from chronic obstructive lung disease is four times higher in the lowest birth weight group, compared against the highest. The observations of Barker's group on chronic obstructive lung disease and birth weight are not entirely surprising, considering growth and development of the respiratory system. Lung development takes place in an orderly sequence, with airways all in place by 16 weeks of gestational age (40 weeks is full term) and about half the adult number of alveoli present at term. Any disruption to the ordered sequence of airway and alveolar development cannot be compensated for later in life. This forms part of

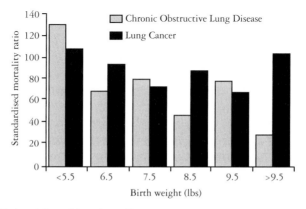

Fig. 11.2 Birth weight and later lung disease.

the 'programming' or 'developmental window' hypothesis, and emphasizes the critical importance of early growth and development for subsequent health and disease. Similar, but more complex hypotheses have been developed for other degenerative diseases including cardio-vascular disease, diabetes and brain development (see Barker 1992).

Establishment of a healthy lifestyle

From birth to full maturity a great deal of growth and some further organ development takes place. For example, lung volume and body weight increase more than 20-fold from birth to adulthood. This growth is fuelled by food intake, and it is not surprising that organ structure is influenced by the quality and constituents of food, as well as its volume. Scotland had the dubious distinction of having the highest incidence of premature death in the developed world due to ischaemic heart disease, and the rest of the UK is not far behind. Although there are multiple genetic and lifestyle factors, including smoking and alcohol consumption, dieting, and behavioral habits acquired in childhood are a cause of subsequent obesity and physical inactivity. A recent report on the Scottish diet identified the high proportion of saturated (animal fat), and low intake of fresh fruit and vegetables as important factors.

Role of parenting

Many of our habits and lifestyles, healthy and otherwise, are established during childhood and adolescence. (Adolescence in this context refers to the psychosocial stage of establishing independence and should not be confused with puberty, which has clearly defined stages of physical/sexual development). The establishment of the smoking habit and dependency on tobacco, for example, is more than twice as likely in children of parents who smoke themselves. Establishment of the exercise habit is more likely in families where the mother takes regular exercise and is less influenced by paternal attitudes to exercise. Parents also have a major influence on the psychosocial development of their children and good parenting is more likely to result in well developed parenting skills in the next generation. Neglect and physical or sexual child abuse are problems that often recur in adults who were exposed as children to these adverse influences.

Late influences: ageing, health, and disease

Normality or abnormality?

The pioneers of geriatric medicine made major advances in their field in the 1930s and 1940s by looking for treatable disease, rather than by carrying out basic research on the ageing process. Even today, for the clinician dealing with older people with illnesses and/or disabilities on a day-to-day basis, there are many practical advantages of an approach that 'looks for treatable disease' and does not delve too deeply into the subtleties of the ageing process. It can, however, be argued that this is a very medical model of life, that it stresses disease, rather than health, and that it tends to ignore the potential for avoiding disease and/or slowing age-related decline.

Compare these two contrasting statements.

Statement 1

It is important to have a good understanding of the normal ageing process because:

1. Physiological changes may affect the way in which disease presents in old age (for example, the increase in heart rate seen in young people in response to exercise, blood loss, or fever may not be evident in older people).

2. Impaired physiological function may affect the susceptibility of an elderly person to disease (for example, immune response may become impaired with age, and this probably explains the increased incidence of tuberculosis and a number of other infections in old age).

3. Once a disease or traumatic event has intervened, age-related homeostatic impairment may hamper recovery (for example, after surgery in older people, fluid depletion or fluid excess may place additional burdens on renal and cardiovascular systems).

4. Drug handling tends to alter with age due to a number of factors, which include impairment in renal and hepatic clearance, and changes in body composition.

5. The reference ranges of laboratory tests or physiological parameters (e.g. target heart rates for exercise programmes) may be affected by age, even where no disease is present.

Statement 2

It is dangerous to place too much emphasis on the normal ageing process because:

1. Over emphasis on age-related decline may lead to attitudes of nihilism among patients and health professionals alike. We should assess the level of function and the presence (or otherwise) of disease in each *individual* person, rather than refer to a table of age-related average values.

2. Treatable disease may be missed by being ascribed simply to 'old age'. The shortness of breath associated with late-onset asthma and the fatigue associated with chronic heart failure are often misdiagnosed as 'just old age'.

Drawing on your own experience and the attitudes of friends, relatives, and professionals whom you have encountered, which of the above arguments is most convincing? How important is a detailed knowledge of normal age-related physiological changes for:

♦ a general practitioner;

♦ a general physician;

♦ a specialist in Medicine for the Elderly;

♦ an architect designing buildings for older people;

♦ an organizer of a 'Keep Fit and Active' Health Promotion campaign aimed at old people;

♦ an organizer of a 'Look Out for Early Signs of Disease' Health Promotion campaign aimed at old people;

♦ a medical student?

Ageism and paternalism

The concept of ageism was introduced by Robert Butler in the 1960s. Writing in 1987 he defined ageism as 'a process of systematic stereotyping and discrimination against people because they are old, just as racism and sexism accomplish this for skin colour and gender'.

A 1994 report from the Medical Research Council concluded 'there is a widespread tendency among health care professionals, purchasers and providers of care to use age as a criterion for the exclusion of older people from certain types of health care'. The report goes on to state that the scientific justification for such exclusions is usually lacking. There is often an important influence of ageing and ageist attitudes on the medical and surgical treatments received by older people.

BOX 2 Ageism in society

Consider the following statements. Do you agree or disagree with them?

1. The portrayal of elderly people in advertising, soap operas, books, plays, and cinema is usually as figures of fun or victims of tragic events.

2. There is so much more disease and disability in elderly people, that it is reasonable to set limits to treatment on the grounds of age alone (e.g. upper age limits for admission to Coronary Care Units).

3. Ageist attitudes (of patients, carers, general public, policy makers, doctors, etc.) are a major problem in disease detection and treatment.

4. In research trials of new drugs, children and elderly people should not be included as they may be unable to give informed consent and they are more likely to have side effects.

BOX 2 Continued

5. In research trials of new drugs, the participation of children and elderly people should be positively encouraged as they are major users and beneficiaries of drugs, and they are more likely to have side effects.

6. If you are discussing details of disease with an old person or a child (particularly if a serious disease is present) you should discuss the details with the family first and get their consent to treatment.

7. The following are ageist: a minimum age for drinking, driving, and sexual activity, a fixed retirement age, the word 'senile' (implying a mixture of confusion and old age), concessionary fares for pensioners, taxation on fuel, separate Departments of Medicine for the Elderly, the words 'elderly', 'old', 'geriatric' (politically correct usage = older people).

8. There should be legislation against ageism, just as there is against race-discrimination and sex-discrimination.

9. As children are non-productive members of society, they have a lesser claim on expensive therapies than do young adults.

10. Old people have a duty to die and get out of the way.

Scope for improvement in health and prevention of disease at different ages

There is a tendency for health promotion campaigns to be targeted at young and middle-aged adults, but this is a restricted (? ageist) view. The importance of establishing healthy lifestyles in children has already been mentioned, but lifestyle changes in old age (difficult though they are to achieve) can also bring significant health gain. A number of body changes such as declining cardiac, renal, and respiratory function and a fall in bone mass, which were previously thought to be an inevitable part of the ageing process may not be inevitable at all. The 'age-related' decline seen in Fig. 11.1 has not always been observed in individuals in long-term studies, particularly when these individuals have had favourable lifestyles and minimal levels of disease.

Physical exercise has been shown to be beneficial in promoting cardiovascular fitness in (a) sedentary teenage girls and (b) men and women after the age of 65 who had never previously done any formal exercise; (c) following acute cardiac disease; and (d) in the presence of chronic lung disease. There is also concern that some young children are getting insufficient exercise ('cot-potatoes', rather than 'couch-potatoes').

Smoking cessation campaigns can also have benefits throughout the age range. Even in old age, further lung damage or arterial disease may be slowed or prevented, and the positive example on the younger generation should not be ignored.

BOX 3 Your conclusions

Look again at the responses you noted to Box 1, Fig. 11.1.

Statement 1

How important is the period of intra-uterine development in determining future health and disease?

Statement 2

How was 'normality' defined in Fig. 11.1? Is it possible to eliminate the effect of disease, environment, and lifestyle in the 'normal' group? Might a change in lifestyle or environment reduce the rate of loss of lung function with age? In trying to predict how an individual will change over his or her lifetime, does it matter that Fig. 11.1 is a cross-sectional study (i.e. at a single point in time), rather than a longitudinal study (i.e. following up individuals for many years)?

Statement 3

In making an initial assessment of an individual whom you have not previously met does it matter that Fig. 11.1 is a cross-sectional study rather than a longitudinal study?

Statement 4

How might smoking and lung disease be related? Think of direct effects and indirect effects (e.g. related to social factors). What about the relative contribution of intra-uterine environment and later environmental/life-style factors. How far can you use data from a cross-sectional study to give health advice to individuals?

Statement 5

In reconsidering Statement 5 ask yourself what 'useful' might refer to. Is the aim to understand the fundamental process of ageing, or to intervene at the population or individual level? Is the intervention aimed at reducing disease, promoting health, improving quality of life, or something else? How easy or difficult is it to modify:

♦ normal development and ageing;

♦ environment and lifestyle;

♦ disease?

Most of all remember that many questions in biological science, sociology and medicine do not have a simple 'yes' or 'no' answer.

Conclusions

Age is therefore shown to have an important influence on many aspects of health. Furthermore, health and its related considerations are important at all ages. A sensitive understanding of the processes and outcomes of development and ageing is important to all health professionals.

SUMMARY POINTS

- In childhood, growing older is something to look forward to, but in late life ageing is not usually viewed so positively!

- Nonetheless, we should avoid stereotyping at any age—for example, some elderly people see old age as the best time of their lives.

- The very young and the very old are similarly vulnerable to instability in body systems (e.g. respiratory, renal, CNS) because the level of reserve function is limited (for different reasons).

- Early development, especially nutrition, early lifestyle, and parenting, has an important effect on health in later life.

- Both the young and the old are vulnerable to discrimination on the grounds of age alone, but ageism—discrimination against the elderly—is probably most prominent.

References and further reading

Barker, D. *et al.* (1991). Relation of birth weight and childhood respiratory illness to adult obstructive lung disease. *British Medical Journal*, **303**, 671–675.

Barker, D.J.P. (1992). *Fetal and Infant Origins of Adult Disease*. British Medical Journal, London.

Evans, J.G. & Williams, T.F. (Eds) (1992). *The Oxford Textbook of Geriatric Medicine*. Oxford University Press, Oxford.

Kramer, M.S. & Joseph, K.S. (1996). Enigma of fetal/infant-origins hypothesis, *Lancet*, **348**, 1254–1255.

Seymour, D.G. & Seymour, R.M. (1989). The physiology of ageing. In: M. S. J. Pathy & P. Finucane (Eds) *Geriatric Medicine, Problems and Practice*. Springer Verlag, Berlin, pp. 1–13.

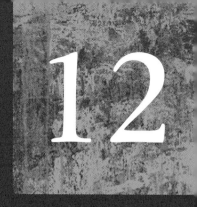

CHAPTER 12

Introduction: illness and healthcare in the community

CHAPTER 12

Introduction: illness and healthcare in the community

In Part 1 we explored the nature of society and the distinction of health from illness. In Part 2 we examined most of the major influences on the health of individuals. In this final Part, we consider ways of reducing the effects of ill health in the community and the contribution that health professionals can make. There is increasing recognition of the importance of Health Promotion (Chapter 13). It makes good sense to try to preserve health and prevent illness, rather than 'locking the stable door after the horse has bolted'. There should be a preventive emphasis all the way through any health care system and, when this is combined with an effective system of primary health care, the result should be a health care system that is not only of high quality, but relatively cheap. Chapter 14 discusses some of the main differences in the way that health care delivery is organized in different countries. Although many might look to the USA as offering the best in health care, the USA compares surprisingly poorly with other countries in terms of overall health outcomes, value for money, and equity. On the other hand, poor countries with a communitarian ethic can produce good results.

In western countries in particular, chronic diseases take up an increasing proportion of health service resources: a point that has been discussed in several earlier chapters. Chapter 15 looks more closely at the characteristics that these chronic disease states have in common. Chapter 16 is concerned with the effects that they may have on an individual's ability to function as a person, look after him or herself, pursue useful employment and enjoy a good social life. Chapter 17 looks specifically at the problem of chronic mental illnesses and vulnerable people like those with learning difficulties or severe personality problems.

It is best to read this section as a whole because, although it is divided into three chapters, the division is artificial as there is considerable overlap between the themes covered in each. Mental, physical and social aspects of chronic illness can never be separated. For example, Chapter 17 highlights older people as a vulnerable section of the community; many of the chronic illnesses described in Chapter 15 are more common in the elderly and degree of disability is often related to age.

Throughout the book there has been a recurring theme of inequity and inequality. A healthcare system that denied or impeded access to some needy individuals because they could not pay (as some systems do) might be regarded as unfair or even unethical. There are, however, more subtle forms of discrimination and inequity many of which have been discussed throughout the book.

In the end, however, death is the great leveller. We therefore end the book (Chapter 18) with a discussion of this very sensitive subject.

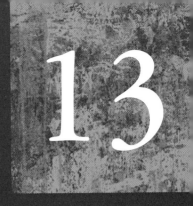

13

CHAPTER 13

Health promotion

CHAPTER 13
Health promotion

Introduction

Health promotion encompasses health education, preventive activities such as screening, and general promotional activities. While there has been a major shift in national and international health policies to promote health in the community through primary care and related services, the avoidance of illness and disease has often been considered a peripheral activity for the NHS.

Recent health policy strategies underline the need for the promotion of health through the combined impact of fiscal policies and the efforts of health care professionals working with patients and community groups. Doctors working in all health care settings are now expected to advise on health behaviours, as well as treat illness symptoms.

In earlier chapters health was defined as a broad concept comprising:

♦ genetic endowment;

♦ access to, and use of, health services at both a primary and secondary level;

♦ the environment: both physical (for example, housing conditions) and social (for example, the composition of your household);

♦ individual behaviour and lifestyle.

Health promotion is largely concerned with the last two points. It seeks to promote a positive health status through a combination of legislation, the provision of preventive services such as immunization, and the development of activities to promote and maintain change to a healthier lifestyle. The actual nature of these activities will vary with the locality in which people reside (urban or rural), their ethnic origins, their socio-economic status, their age, their gender, their household composition, and whether they are in paid employment or not. For example, if you were a government minister concerned with promoting safer sex messages amongst teenagers and young people you might decide to fund:

♦ a national advertising campaign aimed at reaching as many of these age groups as you could—known as a *population approach to health promotion*—together with:

♦ support for the development of projects through local health promotion departments that might develop activities at youth centres with individual young people—an *individual approach to health promotion*. Given the diversity of communities in the UK population local activities will need to reflect religious, cultural and gender differences on attitudes to sex amongst teenagers.

Thus, health promotion may involve a range of agencies (not just health promotion departments), might seek to cover the population or work with groups or individuals, and must be sensitive to differences in behaviour and attitude in a multi-cultural society.

Theories of health education and health promotion

There has always been an information giving aspect to the work of public and community health services, commonly known as health education. Health education is based upon the premise that giving information to individuals might result in a behaviour change or avoidance of a hazard.

Health education is concerned with communication, which might take place in several ways:

♦ education and information about the human body provided for the individual;

♦ information on health and related services and access to these services;

♦ education and information about national, regional and local policies on health.

This approach to promoting health has been criticized as concentrating on individual behaviour and emphasizing what people should not do (for example, don't smoke, don't eat too much fat, don't drink so much), rather than considering the broader factors in the causation of health behaviour patterns.

While there is a role for information, health promotion reflects the wider determinants of health, and the need for policy and practice to enhance health status. Over the last 20 years, a number of approaches to health promotion have evolved. Each of these has a particular emphasis, although these approaches are not mutually exclusive. In this chapter three approaches are considered, namely:

♦ educational;

♦ socio-economic;

♦ psychological.

Educational approach

Strongly linked to health education, this approach seeks to provide knowledge and information, and to develop the necessary skills so that a person can make informed choices about their health. Education in this sense is based upon the assumption that, by increasing knowledge, there will be a change in attitudes that may result in changed behaviour. This approach differs from health education as the information may be delivered using a range of methods, for example, group discussions, workshop sessions, and one-to-one counselling. Much of the work in health promotion departments is based on this approach delivered through a range of activities, such as health fairs, support groups and training courses for professionals who may be working in settings where they can support behaviour change.

Socio-economic approach

This approach is sometimes known as the radical approach as it is based upon the premise that socio-economic status has a direct bearing on health status. Thus, the promotion of positive health status requires a lessening of inequalities in society. The approach has a catch phrase, namely, 'making healthy choices the easy choice'. Achieving the necessary socio-economic changes requires political will and public acceptance of the need for this change. Many of the people who consult doctors live in low-income households and may be unemployed. In this approach national and regional policies to enhance employment opportunities, and to re-distribute income, may do more to enhance quality of life than the mere provision of information on health behaviour. Increasing the income of poor households may do more for the health of those household members than increasing the budget of the NHS. Regardless of government policies, health professionals can support individuals, communities, and local government to consider environmental and lifestyle changes to promote health.

Psychological approach

There is a complex relationship between behaviour, knowledge, attitudes and beliefs, and achieving behaviour change. This approach seeks to encourage individuals to adopt healthy lifestyles by optimizing the control they have over their health. Drawing upon a number of psychological theories, for example, theory of reasoned action, social learning theory, health belief model, stages of change (see Boxes 1–4)—activities based on this approach start from the individual's overall attitude to health and their readiness, or otherwise, to change. Particular emphasis is placed upon identifying whether or not an individual is interested and ready to change, and if so, how to support and maintain any change.

BOX 1 Models of behavioural change (1)

The *Theory of Reasoned Action* argues that behaviour is guided by two broad influences:

◆ an individual's attitude towards certain behaviour. Each attitude, in turn consists of a belief (e.g. smoking can cause cancer) and a value attached to that belief (positive or negative) which may be felt strongly or moderately. Individuals may have a number of (conflicting) attitudes towards a certain behaviour.

◆ individuals have perceptions of what others will think of them displaying certain behaviour (so-called 'subjective norms').

These two major elements combine to form an 'intention' to behave in a certain way, which is closely related to the behaviour itself. Thus, the link between attitudes and behaviour is mediated by a number of processes each of which may influence behaviour.

BOX 2 Models of behavioural change (2)

The *Social Learning Theory* argues that behaviour is guided by expected consequences. The more positive these are, the more likely one is to engage in any particular behaviour. This theory also explains the persistence of certain behaviours with negative consequences. For example:

◆ Short-term gratification is greater than the long-term expected harm. Smoking is a classic example of this; the short-term gratification is instant and experienced as better than the nebulous and long-term potential risk of lung cancer. Self-control involves activating and bringing to mind the longer-term consequences of our actions. Self-control or self-regulation is therefore one of the aims of health promotion.

◆ Denial—a smoker who argues that his granny smoked until she was 96. The individual uses one example to offset their own subjective appraisal of the unhealthy consequences of smoking.

BOX 3 Models of behavioural change (3)

The *Health Belief Model* suggests that the likelihood of an individual engaging in a particular action is a function of their perceptions of the relationship between behaviour and illness, their susceptibility to that illness, the seriousness of the illness, and the particular costs and benefits involved in engaging in the particular action. A final influence on the uptake of any behaviour is the presence of *cues to action*—that is, reminders to engage in certain behaviours.

BOX 3 Continued

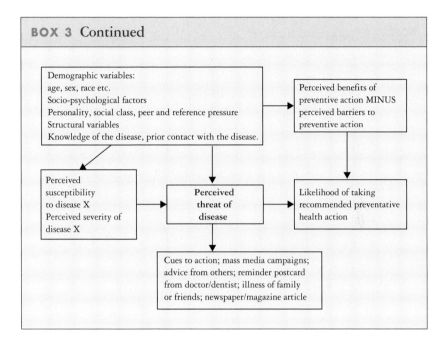

Prevention from a medical perspective

Health can be improved by preventive health care and there are three possible types of intervention:

♦ *Primary prevention* involves measures taken to prevent the onset of illness and injury. It includes efforts to reduce the probability, severity, and duration of future illness and injury, for example, health education directed at encouraging children never to start smoking and immunization.

BOX 4 Models of behavioural change (4)

The stages of change model

Identifies five major stages of change that help explain the move from non-smoking to smoking (i.e. taking up a habit), as well as from smoking to ex-smoking (i.e. giving up smoking under a cessation programme). According to this theory raising awareness about tobacco is a much more appropriate (and successful) intervention for smokers in the precontemplation stage (i.e. when they are considering giving up smoking) than for smokers in the maintenance stage (i.e. the regular smoker). Similarly, intervention aimed at those in the contemplation stage (such as an offer of nicotine patches) will be wasted on those who have not yet reached this stage.

BOX 4 Continued

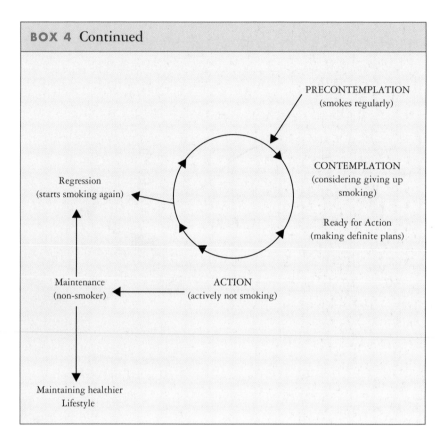

- *Secondary prevention* involves measures to detect pre-symptomatic disease where earlier detection will mean more effective treatment, for example, screening for cervical cancer in women.

- *Tertiary prevention* involves measures to reduce disability from existing illness and to prevent it getting worse, for example, physiotherapy and community support to enhance the quality of life of the chronically ill living at home.

Immunization and screening services are a major component of primary and secondary prevention activities and often take place in primary health care. Activities may be targeted at whole populations (for example, immunization) or at high-risk groups (for example, antenatal tests for pregnant women with a family history of chromosomal abnormality). Prevention, especially screening, is perceived by many health care professionals as a critical component of health promotion in the clinical context. In primary care, GPs often argue that cervical cancer screening services are more relevant to a reduction in morbidity and are more immediately cost effective than running, for example, smoking cessation support groups. Yet smoking status has been implicated in the causation of cervical abnormalities. In summary, work to enhance health status, and prevent illness and disease, must combine activities in a range of health settings and be supported by health, social and public policies.

Health promotion in practice

The World Health Organization (WHO) has promoted health and health promotion, especially through primary health care in its Global Strategy of Health For All:

> 'all people in all countries should have at least such a level of health that they are capable of working productively and of participating actively in the social life of the community in which they live.'

Three main principles to this strategy were identified as:

♦ promotion of lifestyles conducive to health;

♦ prevention of preventable conditions;

♦ rehabilitation and health services.

As a member of the WHO the UK Government has sought to meet the aims of Health For All by developing a series of strategies for the countries of the UK, e.g. 'Towards a Healthier Scotland' (Scottish Executive 1999). This report calls for a 'coherent attack on health inequalities, a special focus on improving children and young people's health, and major initiatives to drive down cancer and heart disease' (see Box 5).

BOX 5 'Towards a Healthier Scotland' main strategies

1. Cross-departmental work in the Scottish Executive with linked action at three levels; first, *life circumstances* that impact on health such as social inclusion, jobs, income, housing, education and environment; secondly, tackling *lifestyles* that lead to illness or early death, for example poor diet, drug misuse, smoking; and thirdly, *prevention* for a number of conditions (such as heart disease, cancers), and to improve child, mental, oral, and sexual health.

2. Public health strategy groups to ensure what are termed *health-friendly policies and initiatives* throughout the Scottish Executive, and promote cross-agency work amongst relevant organizations and professional groups.

3. The funding of four *health demonstration projects* to concentrate on, respectively, young children, responsible sexual behaviour, heart disease, and cancer.

4. On-going *evaluation, monitoring and review* of the strategy with targets set for changes in health behaviours and illnesses to be achieved by 2010.

Similar strategies are being implemented throughout the UK and in Europe. How will health promotion be part of this strategy? The four UK Government agencies responsible for health promotion are developing activities based upon the notion of 'settings' (the workplace, school and hospital) and community development. Activities in the community programme are concerned with the active involvement of people in developing their quality of life based upon issues of importance to them. The settings approach is particularly relevant to medicine as it is likely that doctors may actually be involved on an individual basis as part of an initiative (for example, the NHS health and work programme; Box 6) or invited to provide a professional contribution to a project, for example, an occupational health promotion programme concerned with prevention and coronary heart disease or a project to promote health in schools (Box 7).

BOX 6 The health-promoting hospital

The health-promoting hospital (HPH) movement in Europe originated in the work carried out by members of the Ludwig Bolzmann Institute for Medicine and Medical Sociology at Vienna University. The 1991 Budapest Declaration further defines the basic preconditions necessary for joining the HPH movement as:

> Beyond the assurance of good quality medical services and health care, the health-promoting hospital encourages and supports health-promoting perspectives and activities amongst staff, patients, relatives, visitors and the wider community.

By the early 1990s, 27 countries were members and this includes the UK and Ireland.

For example, in England, the Preston Acute Hospitals Trust have implemented the conditions of the Budapest Declaration through a number of projects:

♦ a healthy environment in a health-promoting hospital;

♦ the management of post-coronary patients;

♦ prevention of accidents;

♦ developing healthy networks and alliances;

♦ health promotion aspects of collecting and disposing of clinical waste.

The Health at work initiative was set up to improve the health of NHS employees by enhancing opportunities for staff to adopt positive health practices. As part of this strategy Southampton University Hospital Trust introduced a £50 incentive to encourage staff to swap cars for alternative forms of transport. Since the introduction of the scheme cycling among staff has increased by 70%.

BOX 7 The health-promoting school

The concept of the health-promoting school recognizes that health education does not only exist through the taught curriculum, but is intensified by the supportive interest of school, home, and community. Work in the classroom may be supported and reinforced by:

♦ the values and attitudes implicit in the organization, policies, and staffing of schools;

♦ closer links with parents and families;

♦ closer liaison and interaction between the school and the community;

♦ a supportive political and legislative 'environment'.

Example: the Hackney well-being in schools project

This action research project aims to develop mental health promotion for young people in Hackney (London) schools. Steered by a multi-professional group working alongside pupils, it is promoting a whole-school approach to enhancing self-esteem and confidence premised upon a model of empowerment. It has focused upon the specific needs of girls, approaches to anti-bullying, improving positive image, and developing appropriate personal and social health education.

Evaluating health promotion

The success of health promotion activities is difficult to gauge, because of the long-term nature of most of the outcomes and the difficulty of measuring these. Yet it is important to make some attempts if we are to justify the input of financial and human resources. However, even with the most rigorously evaluated and appropriate health promotion package, it is impossible to achieve total success in effecting health behavioural change. Ultimately, it is for individuals to decide, and the limit of the health professional's duty is probably to ensure that individual choice is as well-informed and well-facilitated as possible.

SUMMARY POINTS

♦ Health promotion includes health education, preventative activities such as screening, and general promotional activities.

♦ Recent UK government health strategies emphasize the need for promotion of health through the combined impact of public policy and community based work by health professionals, i.e. a combination of population- and individual-based approaches.

> ### SUMMARY POINTS Continued
>
> ◆ The principal approaches of health promotion overlap, but are usually (a) educational, (b) socio-economic, or (c) psychological.
>
> ◆ The main medical approaches are through preventive health care, which may be primary, secondary, or tertiary in terms of level of intervention.
>
> ◆ Behavioural change depends on a number of factors within the person, as well as in the person's immediate, and wider social and cultural environment.
>
> ◆ Integrated projects, such as health-promoting hospitals and schools, offer perhaps the most promising way ahead for health promotion.

References and further reading

Acheson, D. (1998). *Independent Inquiry into Inequalities in Health Report*, The Acheson Report). Stationery Office, London.

Catford, J. (1993). Auditing health promotion: what are the vital signs of quality? *Health Promotion International*, 8, 67–68.

Downie, R., Fyfe, C. & Tannahill, A. (1990). *Health Promotion. Models and Values*. Oxford Medical Publications, Oxford.

Naidoo, J. & Wills, J. (1998). *Practising Health Promotion. Dilemmas and Challenges*. Bailliere Tindall, London.

Prochaska, J.O. & DiClemente, C. (1984). *The Transtheoretical Approach: crossing traditional foundations of change*. Don Jones/Irwin, Harnewood.

Scottish Executive (1999). *Towards a Healthier Scotland*. Department of Health, Scottish Office, Edinburgh.

Scriven, A. & Orme, J. (Eds) (1996). *Health Promotion. Professional Perspectives*, Macmillan, London.

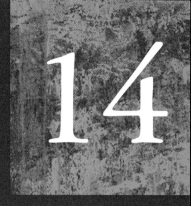

CHAPTER 14

Organization of medical care

CHAPTER 14

Organization of medical care

Healthcare systems: international comparisons

The ways that countries differ in how medical care is delivered to their populations is principally to do with differences in organization of primary medical care and general practice, rather than hospital and specialist care (Table 14.1). At one end of the spectrum, patients could simply go direct to specialists when they thought they required them. Soviet Russia used to have the nearest to this kind of system, with health care, in cities at least, provided directly by huge polyclinics, staffed entirely by specialists. The main problems with this direct kind of system are that the patient needs to know which specialist to select and, if he or she has a problem that involves different body systems or a number of different problems, s/he may need to see a number of different specialists. In countries like the USA, there is a hybrid system where, although patients increasingly consult nurse practitioners or primary care physicians, they may also directly consult specialists or go direct to the emergency room of a hospital. At the other end of the spectrum is the UK system of medical care through the National Health Service (NHS), where it is generally not possible for the patient to see a specialist without first consulting a general practitioner (GP). The GP acts primarily as their personal medical advisor, much akin to legal and financial advisers, in this sense. Of course, referral to specialist care is only a small part of the GP's job—nine out of 10 illnesses are treated within the practice, without specialist referral—but this 'gatekeeper' role of the general practitioner is now generally acknowledged to be an important component of efficient health care delivery.

Another, related, issue is how best to fund comprehensive health care for a population. Since its inception, the aim of the UK National Health Service has

Table 14.1 Characteristics of health care systems

System	Characteristics	Example
Totalitarian/Marxist	State provided and state owned. Staff wholly employed and staff costs generally low; private practice illegal; no direct payments.	Former Soviet Union, Cuba
Communitarian/ National Health Service	State provided and publicly owned. Most staff directly employed (except general practitioners). Public care dominant, but private practice allowed	United Kingdom
Insurance/ Social Security	Health is a consumer service, but guaranteed by compulsory insurance. Doctors largely self-employed entrepreneurs. Mixed private and public ownership of facilities. Payments for services mostly indirect	France, Germany
Libertarian/ pluralistic	Doctors are self-employed entrepreneurs. Private provision dominates with public care providing only a 'safety net' for disadvantaged groups.	United States of America
Entrepreneurial/ unregulated	No system of state intervention in personal health care (although there may be public health programmes) so that health care is entirely like any other consumer item	Some African, Asian and Latin American countries

been to provide all necessary health care for everyone in the country, regardless of means and free at the point of need. One problem has been that as medicine becomes more technical and expensive (e.g. coronary artery by-pass grafts for heart disease), and as people become more educated and assertive, public expectation of what the NHS should be able to provide has risen progressively. At the same time it is not widely appreciated that the USA government spends just as much on public provision of health care as does the UK government (Table 14.2), but gets much less for its money. In the USA public health care covers only the very elderly and the poor. The USA's health care system is

Table 14.2 Total health expenditure

Country	$ per person p.a. (1997)	% of total expenditure publicly funded
USA	3925	46.4
Canada	2095	71.4
UK	1347	84.3

National Centre for Health Statistics (1999).

mostly privately funded by individuals themselves and their employers, through medical insurance schemes. Altogether health care costs the USA almost three times as much as it does the UK.

World Health Report 2000 (WHO)

There is a general consensus in the UK that greater investment in public health care is the most efficient way forward. A recent report of the World Health Organization (WHO) tends to support this view. For the first time it analyses health services in terms of efficiency of delivery of health care (so far as is possible). For example, it is obvious that Sweden enjoys better health than Uganda—life expectancy in Sweden is almost twice as long as in Uganda—but Sweden spends 35 times as much *per capita* on its health system. On the other hand, Pakistan spends almost precisely the same amount per person on health care as Uganda, out of an income per person that is close to Uganda's, but it has a life expectancy almost 25 years higher. The crucial comparison is 'like with like'—why are health outcomes in Pakistan so much better than in Uganda, for the same expenditure?

> And it is health expenditure that matters, not the country's total income, because one society may choose to spend less of a given income on health than another. Each health system should be judged according to the resources actually at its disposal, not according to other resources which in principle could have been devoted to health but were used for something else. (WHO 2000)

In summary, WHO asserts that health systems have a responsibility not just to improve people's health, but to protect them against the financial cost of illness—and to treat them with dignity. The report charges health systems with three fundamental objectives:

- *Health:* this means making the health status of the entire population as good as possible over people's whole life cycle, taking account of both premature mortality and disability. The WHO measurement of disability-adjusted life expectancy (DALE), takes account of the burden of disease—the number of 'disability-adjusted life years' (DALYs) lost. This has the advantage of being directly comparable with life expectancy estimated from mortality alone and is readily comparable across populations.

♦ *Responsiveness:* is a measure of how a system meets people's social expectations of how they should be dealt with. For example, prior to 1990, for all that the Soviet medical system might have been relatively effective from a medical point of view, it had become highly impersonal and inhumane in the way that it processed people. 'A common complaint in many countries about public sector health workers focuses on their rudeness and arrogance in relations with patients' (WHO 2000).

♦ *Fair financing:* this means that individuals should be protected against catastrophic financial loss due to illness. A fairly financed system ensures that the costs of illness are distributed according to ability to pay, rather than to the risk of illness. 'A health system in which individuals are sometimes forced into poverty through their purchase of needed care, or forced to do without it because of the cost, is unfair' (WHO 2000). For this reason, direct 'out of pocket' financing systems are generally regressive and the ideal is to 'disconnect a household's financial contribution to the health system from its health risks' largely through prepayment schemes and subsidies from general taxation. The concept of 'pooling' of risk is central: prepayment (e.g. insurance) systems that discriminate against high-risk clients are inhumane and unethical (see Fig. 14.1). Another

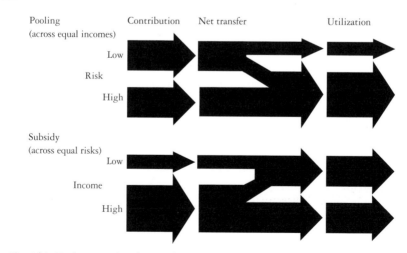

Fig. 14.1 Pooling to redistribute risk and cross-subsidy for greater equity (arrows indicate flow of funds.

Source: The WHO Report (2000).

major factor in underdeveloped countries is that they may not have adequate administrative systems for the collection of central revenues and so are forced to depend more on direct payments. (For example, whilst general taxation on average accounts for more than 40% of Gross Domestic Product (GDP) in developed countries, it accounts for less than 20% in low-income countries. These countries depend more on an informal ('black') economy.

The methods used by WHO to measure these objectives (health status, responsiveness, and fair financing) are detailed in the report (WHO 2000) and combined to produce a ranking of the health systems of different countries. This novel classification of the success of different ways of organizing health systems results in a rank order, which is in many ways surprising (Table 14.3).

Table 14.3 WHO's rating of health care systems

The top 40 rated countries				The bottom 40 rated countries			
1	France	21	Belgium	152	Togo	172	Rwanda
2	Italy	22	Colombia	153	Turkmenistan	173	Afghanistan
3	San Marino	23	Sweden	154	Tajikistan	174	Cambodia
4	Andorra	24	Cyprus	155	Zimbabwe	175	South Africa
5	Malta	25	Germany	156	Tanzania	176	Guinea-Bissau
6	Singapore	26	Saudi Arabia	157	Djibouti	177	Swaziland
7	Spain	27	United Arab Emirates	158	Eritrea	178	Chad
8	Oman	28	Israel	159	Madagascar	179	Somalia
9	Austria	29	Morocco	160	Vietnam	180	Ethiopia
10	Japan	30	Canada	161	Guinea	181	Angola
11	Norway	31	Finland	162	Mauritania	182	Zambia
12	Portugal	32	Australia	163	Mali	183	Lesotho
13	Monaco	33	Chile	164	Cameroon	184	Mozambique
14	Greece	34	Denmark	165	Laos	185	Malawi
15	Iceland	35	Dominica	166	Congo	186	Liberia
16	Luxemburg	36	Costa Rica	167	North Korea	187	Nigeria
17	Netherlands	37	USA	168	Namibia	188	Congo Republic
18	United Kingdom	38	Slovenia	169	Botswana	189	Central African Republic
19	Ireland	39	Cuba	170	Niger	190	Burma
20	Switzerland	40	Brunei	171	Equatorial Guinea	191	Sierra Leone

The WHO report judged each country's health system against the most that it estimated could be achieved with its level of health service expenditure. Thus, it was possible for a relatively poor country to achieve a better result than a comparatively rich one.

Horizontal and vertical equity

The WHO report puts a cogent argument that governments should protect people against financial risk in matters of health, whether the system is publicly or privately financed. This means that the overall system should ideally provide both horizontal equity (treating alike all who face the same health need) and vertical equity (treating preferentially those with the greatest needs):

> And it should assure not only that the healthy subsidise the sick, as any prepayment arrangement will do in part, but also that the burden of financing is fairly shared by having the better-off subsidise the less well-off. This generally requires spending public funds in favour of the poor. (WHO 2000)

Private systems will tend not to cover well services that have large externalities; that is, situations where there are public health, rather than identifiable individual, benefits. Good examples are communicable disease control and public health environmental measures. Private demand for such measures may be low, but they may have large health benefits. Differences in centrally funded public health programmes account for much of the differences in health indices between countries with comparable levels of overall health expenditure (e.g. the difference between Pakistan and Uganda, referred to earlier).

This leads to the question of what is the 'bottom line'? How should countries prioritize their provision of health care? Rationing of health care is difficult, always controversial, yet necessary for the fundamental functioning of any system with limited resources (Fig. 14.2).

The concept of quality adjusted life years (QALY) provides one method of aiding decision-making. It was devised in the 1970s by the US Office of Technology Assessment to provide a balance of the *quantity* of life, measured in years and *quality* of life in these years. It can be used to estimate and compare the results of different treatments and medical interventions. Table 14.4 shows the results of some of these calculations for the UK.

Deployment of resources

One of the striking things is how differently countries deploy resources. The WHO report employs a novel way of demonstrating this (Fig.14.3).

Figure 14.3 compares the relative and absolute levels of spending on different attributes of healthcare systems in four different countries. It provides a measure of the perceived importance of each of these attributes to each system. The figure illustrates how the USA is close to the maximum for every input.

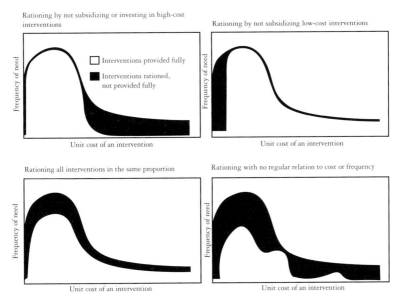

Fig. 14.2 Different ways of rationing health interventions according to cost and frequency of need.

Source: The WHO Report (2000).

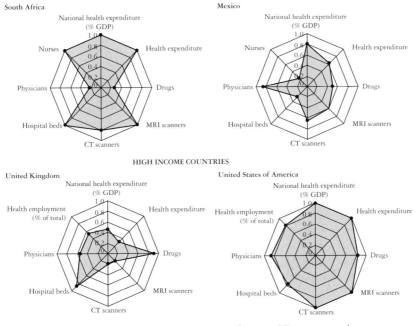

Fig. 14.3 Health systems input mix: comparison of two middle income and two high-income countries.

Note: Data are presented as fractions of the maximum value (among the pairs of countries shown) for each individual indicator: these maximum values define the 'frontier' inside which all the data lie. All indicators are per capita except for total National health expenditure and health employment.

Source: The WHO Report (2000).

Table 14.4 Quality adjusted life year (QALY) of competing therapies: some tentative estimates

	Cost/QALY (£ August 1990)
Cholesterol testing and diet therapy only (all adults, aged 40–69)	220
Neurological intervention for head injury	240
GP advice to stop smoking	270
Anti-hypertensive therapy to prevent stroke (ages 35–64)	940
Pacemaker implantation	1100
Hip joint replacement	1180
Coronary artery bypass graft (left main vessel disease, severe angina)	2090
Kidney transplant	4710
Breast cancer screening	5780
Heart transplantation	7840
Coronary artery bypass graft (single vessel disease, moderate angina)	19,870
Erythropoietin treatment for anaemia in dialysis (assuming a 10% reduction in mortality)	107,780
Neurosurgical interventions for malignant intracranial tumours	126,290

Adapted from Maynard (1994).

It is an early adopter of every new medical technology and it pays the price for that, in that the population of the USA pays through taxation and health insurance a larger share of the global costs in developing new technology than do those of other countries. Countries like UK (and Sweden and Denmark, not shown here) wait until the technology has been established and has come down in price! USA (and to an extent Canada) come out relatively poorly in the WHO stakes, compared with UK and the Nordic countries, and this is part of the reason.

The WHO report concludes that it is possible for quite poor countries to achieve considerable health equality, respect for persons and financial fairness, and that, conversely, there can be much waste of resources in rich countries, such as the USA, which do not achieve nearly as much as they might with the highest per capita spending on health care in the world. UK lies somewhat between the two, but has no cause to be complacent. There is always room for improvement!

Primary healthcare in the United Kingdom

The UK NHS strives to meet the WHO criteria by providing an equitable system of health care for all of its population, still mainly free at the point of use. Health services in the UK today have to deal less with acute infective disease and more with the consequences of chronic disease. This has required the development of new services and the constant re-organization of care. Some diseases that were previously associated with a high degree of mortality now result in more morbidity in the community because of a higher proportion of disabled survivors in the community. In the past, many chronic diseases were managed mainly by the hospital sector. Today, an increasing proportion of these patients is becoming the responsibility of healthcare professionals working in primary care. This shift in the place of care has partly contributed to the huge increase in general practice workload in the past three decades. Another factor has been the central role that the primary care team has been given in co-ordinating a number of preventive services, such as childhood immunization and cervical cancer screening. Technological advances, professional development, patient preferences for local-based services, and governmental desires to constrain healthcare costs will continue to drive the shift of much healthcare from secondary to primary care.

It is widely acknowledged that the relative success of the NHS (in the WHO tables UK is 18th against USA's 37th place) is due to its focus on primary care (Starfield 1992), especially bringing different health professionals together in primary health care teams. Table 14.5 lists the main professionals consistently involved, but other professional groups may function as occasional members of the team, or may in the future play a more major role. These include clinical psychologists, community psychiatric nurses (CPNs), specialist outreach nurses (e.g. stoma care and care of cancer patients), qualified counsellors, and social workers.

It is difficult for small units to provide the range and quality of service that is increasingly expected of primary care, and practices are forming into larger and larger units. The average practice size is probably around about five or six doctors in the UK, but there are some practices with 20 doctors or more. The average 'list size' or number of people registered for NHS care is about 1800 people per doctor (rather less in Scotland and in rural areas generally). The concept of the 'registered list' is central to UK general practice. It means that the practice covers a defined subset of the population, whether they are well or ill. Although most of the work of a practice tends to be with the relatively small minority of the practice population who are ill, there is an increasing emphasis on health promotion in the practice population as a whole, including those 'well' persons who might not spontaneously seek medical advice.

Recent trends are towards a more corporate model for primary health care with already fairly large general practices aligned together on a mainly geographical

Table 14.5 The primary care team (PCT)

Title	Qualifications	Employed by	Brief description of role
General Practioner (GP)	Medical degree, with several years of specific postgraduate training and vocational accreditation	Self-employed	Provision of routine medical care and preventive activities. Referrals to others in the PCT, and to secondary care. Director of the practice, which is a small business
Practice (treatment room) nurse	Fully registered nurse often with additional training	General practice	Works on the practice premises alongside the doctors. Does a variety of diagnostic and treatment procedures
District nurse (DN)	Fully registered nurse with additional training	Local health authority	Has his or her own independent work, but is also 'attached' to practice(s) and liaises with them
Health visitor (HV)	Fully registered nurse with several levels of additional training	Local health authority	Position similar to DN, but works more in the field of prevention, health promotion and public health
Midwife	As DN and HV with specific training in midwifery	Local health authority	Entirely responsible for their own caseload of pregnant women, but liase with general practice
Receptionist	May have no formal training although most have now attended local courses	General practice	Reception and administrative responsibilities (e.g. filing). Should not undertake any medical tasks as they are not trained for this
Medical secretary	May have some specific training in medical work in addition to basic secretarial training	General practice	Preparation of correspondence, etc.
Pharmacist	Graduate level education and further training	Self-employed/ local health authority	Local ('community') pharmacists are variably involved with general practice. Some health centres house their own pharmacy. At another level health authorities employ pharmacists to provide general advice to groups of practices

basis for administrative and organizational purposes, including allocation of resources (e.g. budgets for prescribing) and clinical accountability and quality control ('clinical governance'). In England and Wales, these larger administrative units may be Primary Care Groups (PCGs) or more formally constituted Primary Care Trusts (PCTs). In Scotland, the larger units, known as Local Health Care Cooperatives (LHCCs), have a more advisory role, with all regions having Primary Health Care Trusts (PHCTs) to operate financial budgets. Furthermore, emergency medical care at evenings and weekends is increasingly provided by groups of GPs functioning together as out-of-hours co-operatives.

Before they consult doctors, most people have already obtained advice from relatives or friends or from professional advisers such as nurses, health visitors and pharmacists. NHS Direct, in which the public can call 24-h telephone advice lines staffed by specially trained nursing staff, is a new kind of service that develops and formalizes this 'pre-medical' level of advice, and which complements the medical service provided by general practitioners.

Finally, there has been greater recent emphasis on consumer responsiveness and public involvement in health service governance. The main ways in which this is achieved are through elected Community Health Councils, patient representatives at all levels of organization, including the practice, and easier and less formal methods for presentation and investigation of complaints about clinical and other services.

Other community-based services

Local government authorities and Departments of Public Health are responsible for direct provision of other community-based health services, such as school nurses and doctors, and community child health specialists (who are mainly responsible for children with disability and handicap), and such matters as environmental safety and infectious diseases control where they will liase closely with other departments such as the Health and Safety Inspectorate. Local Authorities are also responsible for the licensing and general oversight of institutions such as homes for the elderly, and for the provision of domestic help for the elderly and others living at home (Home Help Service). These services are not necessarily provided free of charge.

SUMMARY POINTS

- ◆ Hospitals throughout the world are broadly similar in the way that they deliver medical care. There is much greater variation between countries in how primary care is organized.
- ◆ A good system of primary care is an essential component of an efficient and equitable health care system.

SUMMARY POINTS Continued

- Wealthy countries like USA may waste money on health care, whilst much poorer countries may provide good health care systems.

- Systems that deprive people of needed care or bankrupt them because of it are unethical. 'Pooling of risk' is a primary feature of an ethical system.

- The overall resource that each country has for health care needs to be wisely spent, with an inevitable degree of rationing.

- The structure of Primary Health Care Teams (PHCT) in the UK is briefly described.

References and further reading

Maynard, A. (1994). Prioritising health care—dreams and reality. In: M. Malek (Ed.) *Setting Priorities in Health Care*. Wiley, Chichester.

National Centre for Health Statistics (1999). *Health, United States, 1999 with Health and Ageing Chartbook*, NCHS, Hyattsville.

Starfield, B. (1992). *Primary Care: concept, evaluation, and policy*. Oxford University Press, Oxford.

World Health Organization (2000). *The World Health Report 2000. Health Systems: improving performance*. World Health Organization, Geneva.

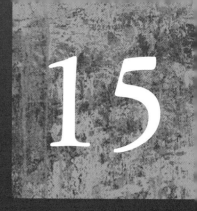

15

CHAPTER 15
Chronic illness

CHAPTER 15
Chronic illness

When illness cannot be cured

Introduction

One of the biggest changes that has occurred in the practice of medicine since the first half of the twentieth century has been an increase in the importance of chronic diseases. Essentially, an acute illness (such as tonsillitis) is one with a defined start and end-point (usually with little time between these) and is often susceptible to cure. A chronic illness often has an insidious onset, rarely has a cure, and consequently lasts for years or a lifetime.

Modern medicine has been able to cure many of the scourges of earlier days. Sanitation, antibiotics, and immunization programmes have cured, emasculated, or even eradicated diseases such as pneumonia, tuberculosis, and smallpox, at least in Western countries. Infant mortality has declined and life expectancy increased continuously in these countries. However, with the demise of infectious diseases has come the emergence of chronic and degenerative disorders, such as cancer and osteoarthritis, ischaemic heart disease, and the respiratory diseases. These tend to be diseases for which no cure is available or which affect particularly older age groups within an ageing society. There is not (at least yet) the equivalent of an antibiotic to treat these, so our attention is drawn towards their prevention and control. Most of them have multi-factorial origin and effects, and there may never be, therefore, a cure as radical as those which secured the public health revolution of the twentieth century.

Persistent diseases that do not lead to early death therefore constitute an important group of health problems. Sufferers may endure multiple handicaps that affect physical, social, and psychological well-being. Constraints on family life, failure to re-establish the functional capacity to work and unremitting physical discomfort, or chronic pain, are all commonplace facts of life for patients with chronic disease. This chapter aims to extend your understanding and insight into a number of facets of these diseases. Think of people or families you know, where there has been a chronic illness. This might be something obvious, such as rheumatoid arthritis, something less obvious, such as diabetes, or covert, such as inactive multiple sclerosis or epilepsy. Consider the consequences of chronic disease on the individual and his or her immediate family. Consider also the facilities available to help those with chronic disease.

Epidemiology

A chronic disease is one that continues for a relatively long time, or is so frequently recurring or relapsing, that its effects on health are virtually continuous (Fig. 15.1).

The epidemiology of chronic illness is not straightforward. The incidence (i.e. number of new cases) may be difficult to assess as the onset is often insidious or not obvious. In many examples there is a spectrum of disease activity and the point at which one is classified as a case is arbitrary, often depending upon individual 'symptom thresholds', or other cultural or medical factors. The prevalence (i.e. number of existing cases) may be difficult to assess as the disease may follow a variable course, including changes in severity, remission (i.e. temporary abatement), relapse, recovery, and recurrence. Nonetheless, it is important to have some indicators of both incidence and prevalence to inform both consulting room discussions and health service planning. In general, as opposed to acute diseases, chronic diseases have a low incidence and a relatively high prevalence (See also Chapter 3.).

Local health authorities will wish to know the incidence of new clinical events in order to ensure that there are services capable of coping with the immediate care for the purposes of diagnosis and early treatment. Social services will be more interested in the overall prevalence, not necessarily of disease, but of particular types of disability, in order that they can ensure that appropriate provision is made within the community.

Health-care economists may be interested in these, but also in the total effect, looking at the impact on national resources of disability of various types. There will be consequences for the individual who has the disease, disability, and handicap, their family, their local medical, and social services, but also an

Condition	Estimated prevalence per 100,000 population
Osteoarthritis	12,890–29,000
Rheumatoid arthritis	1000–2500
Ischaemic heart disease	2000–not known
Chronic obstructive airways disease	1800–8000
Stroke (survivors)	550–1000
Epilepsy	300–500
Cerebral palsy	200
Traumatic brain disease	150
Parkinsonism	110–200
Stomas	70–160
Multiple sclerosis	80–100
Spinal injury	14
Muscular dystrophy	10–20
Huntington's chorea	10
Motor neuron disease	5–10

Fig. 15.1 Prevalence of some examples of chronic disease.

impact on national economy in terms of the size of the working population and the need to financially support those who are no longer able to contribute positively to the economic future of a nation.

Aetiology/development of chronic disease

Chronicity does not arise simply because current medical knowledge is unable to treat some disease pathologies completely. A chronic disease is not simply an acute disease that has lasted for a long time, but is the long-term outcome of a complex interaction of factors.

The causes of most chronic diseases are unknown. In a few instances there is a clear genetic factor, for instance, in haemophilia. For many chronic diseases, however, there is probably a genetic predisposition that may then be influenced by an environmental component, e.g. asthma and diabetes. In a few instances, a disease may be almost entirely environmental, e.g. asbestosis.

Until we understand more about the fundamental causes of chronic diseases it is often difficult to unravel these various influences. However, it is evident that some diseases have more than one individual in a family who may be affected. Under those circumstances there can be considerable anxieties, such as 'will I end up like my brother', 'will I pass this onto my child', or 'have I caught this from somebody else in the family?' The latter can be a particular anxiety in sexually transmitted disease, such as HIV infection resulting in AIDS. Anxieties of this type are further influenced if one member of a family is very severely affected. However, it is not always the case that others will be so severely affected or have the same manifestations. Even in diseases with a strong genetic component individuals can differ in the development and severity of the disease.

Vulnerability

An individual's capacity to resist disease, to repair damage, and restore normal physiological homeostasis is referred to loosely as 'vulnerability'. This concept tends to be used in the context of an acute episode of illness. Similar factors can contribute importantly to the persistence of disease and therefore to chronic illness. They are of particular importance at the extremes of life. Most organs of the body have a reserve capacity, i.e. more than is needed for even maximal function, but this reserve capacity is not fully developed in the newborn and declines greatly in most elderly people. Vulnerability is further explored in Chapter 16.

Figure 15.2 shows schematically the relationship between such hypothetical functional reserve, symptom threshold, and ageing. Certain organs, such as the liver, retain a considerable capacity to restore function following injuries, whereas others such as the brain are much more limited. The concept of the functional reserve of an organ helps understand why some individuals are more susceptible to chronic illness than others. Healthy organs develop in healthy

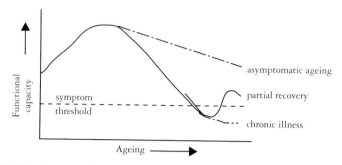

Fig. 15.2 The relationship between functional capacity, symptom threshold, and ageing.

environments; maintenance of adequate nutrition, relative freedom from disease, and the adaptive demands of repeated external stresses can all promote increased functional reserve capacity. It is not surprising that socio-economic deprivation (sometimes associated with premature parental death), hardship, and endemic infections can singly or together make the persistence of a disease more likely. It is perhaps not so obvious that psychological adaptive factors, sometimes acquired early in life, can also contribute to the likelihood of chronicity. The following case illustrates how this might arise.

CASE 1 Angela Barron

Angela's father suffered a sudden and fatal heart attack aged 44, when Angela was 7 years old. An only child, she was the focus of her mother's consuming attention. Unlike other children, she was rarely allowed to play unsupervised and was frequently excused games on insubstantial grounds. Secure in her mother's affections and a model pupil she easily qualified for university. In her first term, before her first tutorial she became increasingly anxious, feeling unprepared, and inadequate. Complaining of palpitations, uncomfortable abdominal, and chest sensations she sought reassurance from a local general practitioner. This was rapidly effective, but the symptoms soon recurred. Later presentations included more complex symptoms, some suggestive of early heart disease. She was advised that her family history placed her at increased risk and that investigations as a hospital in-patient were merited. Although signs of heart disease could not be detected, the admission provided an opportunity for investigations of bowel function. On discharge from hospital her bowel symptoms worsened (she suffered persistent diarrhoea) and she developed new menstrual symptoms. Re-admission led to laparoscopy and the detection of an 'ovarian cyst'. Frequent absences from college led to academic failure, poor work record, and frequent attendances at her family doctor. By age 30 she was described as 'miserable, socially isolated and repeatedly requesting pain killers'.

Angela Barron had an over-protective mother who did not prepare her sufficiently for adult independence. Initial effective reassurance rapidly reduced her anxiety (and its somatic correlates), but probably encouraged her to seek medical reassurance too easily. Her family history seemed sufficient to warrant investigation, but this, in turn, increased her dependency on medical support. New symptoms developed and strengthened her use of symptom formation, consultation, and investigation as a means to control her own internal feelings. Such a process of chronic somatization can follow the onset of most types of disease pathology in vulnerable individuals, and sometimes arises in the absence of any disease pathology at all.

Obvious individual differences in the setting of symptom thresholds are due to factors such as age or knowledge about bodily functions. However, some differences are much less obvious, such as the psychological processes an individual may bring to bear on the recognition of an altered bodily sensation. For example, a woman with a family history of fatal breast cancer may surprisingly choose to ignore or deny breast changes that are present, and not seek investigation for fear of what she might learn. More complex examples can include hard-working, competitive individuals who set and achieve high personal goals attained sometimes at the expense of the feelings of others. For such people, private or public recognition of frailty can be seen as an unacceptable weakness, to be denied at all costs. Symptom thresholds in those individuals, often possessed of a high personal commitment to the control of feelings, can be set at levels that further jeopardize their health.

Artificially high symptom thresholds, when crossed, can have consequences that appear catastrophic for the individual, quite out of proportion with the nature or extent of the pathological process as illustrated by the following case.

CASE 2 Colin Duncan

At school, Colin had been a star athlete. His precocious physical development gave him exceptional speed and strength, and led to many representative honours. He trained and studied hard to the exclusion of any other pastime or interest. His younger sister was receiving chemotherapy meanwhile, in treatment of leukaemia. His family did not discuss his sister's illness with him, feeling that he should not be distracted from fulfilment of his ambition. Months later, recovering at home from flu he realized how ill his sister had become, and did not return to training, complaining instead of persistent 'flu-like symptoms'. He lost considerable performance ability and avoided competition, preferring to spend time with his sister. He complained of persistent tiredness, easy fatigue, poor concentration, and difficulty in sleeping. He attributed this to the earlier viral infection.

Mental mechanisms can contribute substantially to the persistence of some symptoms. Although these can appear to be primarily somatic in nature, sometimes primary psychological processes are thought to be causal. Occasionally, individuals appear not to be able to describe their own mental lives in anything other than somatic terms. Colin and probably his family had gained a great deal from his sporting achievements. His success had, however, been achieved at some personal cost. Even once Colin had acknowledged this he was unable to accommodate both his feelings for his sister and his needs to achieve sporting excellence, other than by reporting persistent somatic symptoms.

Impact of chronic illness

If you have known or visited a chronically ill individual in their home environment you will appreciate that chronic disease in individuals has wide reaching implications for the individual, their immediate family, their neighbours, friends, the community in which they live, and the nation as a whole.

Individuals

Individuals vary considerably in their response to the development of a chronic disease. There may be a period of denial, the question of 'why me', self-pity, blaming others, giving in totally (see Chapter 10). All these reactions are very common and understandable. Some, however, if they persist as a major response to chronic disease, do not positively assist the individual in coping with the consequences. On the other hand, development of disease in an individual may give a positive purpose to their life; for instance, a hitherto very self-centred individual, who develops a devastating illness that is incurable, and then suddenly becomes the driving force behind fund-raising for research into the disease or to support their local self-help group, hospital, or hospital department.

Family

The occurrence of chronic disease in a family can have deep and far-reaching effects. These may include the effects of reduced (or lost) income, and a reduced contribution to the running of the family and household. There are often significant demands on financial, emotional, and temporal resources from the need to nurse and care for the family member, and attend hospitals and clinics. This is often at the expense of other family members' work, leisure, and health. There is a higher prevalence of chronic illness in families where one member has a chronic disease. There is also a higher rate of marital separation and emotional problems such as depression. These problems may go unrecognized or unattended, because of the obvious needs of the individual with the initial disease.

Community/society

Many of these implications may extend to the community, if neighbours, friends, and relatives are involved in caring. A well-organized community may respond by helping with things like transport, shopping, and visiting, and these are important in maintaining maximal health. Alternatively, in a less supportive community, a chronic illness may isolate an individual, leading to deteriorating general health and well-being. One of the ways of judging the success of a community is the way in which it looks after its infirm members. This, of course, requires a contribution to the community in times of health, and this contribution will often be one of the casualties after development of a chronic illness.

Natural history of chronic illness

Variable course of disease (see Table 15.1)

Different diseases behave differently over time:

◆ Some may have an acute onset such as in stroke or myocardial infarction. The immediate symptoms may be very severe, but with some recovery to a greater or lesser extent, leading to a persistent impairment, but a stable one. Sometimes the improvement is such that the individual has no impairment. The pathological process, however, is still there.

◆ In other instances, the onset may be gradual with a steady, slow, or more rapid deterioration. This is often the case in angina, where there is a gradual reduction in the distance an individual can walk before the onset of chest pain.

◆ There may, on the other hand, be relapse and remission. An individual who has had a stroke may recover very well only to suffer a further stroke. There is one type of multiple sclerosis in which there is relapse and remission as a natural consequence of the disease. Patients with cancer may go into remission with treatment, but the disease relapses again later.

◆ Some disease states may not cause a great deal of initial disability, but as complications arise disabilities appear. For instance, in diabetes there may

Table 15.1 Variable course of disease

Acute onset	Recovery
	Stable
	Progressive
Gradual onset	Recovery
	Stable
	Progressive
Relapse and remission	

be no disability at first, with only some restrictions in diet required. If, however, the individual suffers complications, such as renal disease or eye disease, additional impairments, disabilities, and handicaps will appear, and more treatment will be required.

♦ Within the same disease the course may vary. For example, a person may suffer one or two episodes of neurological loss associated with multiple sclerosis and never have further trouble. Some patients with multiple sclerosis will have a disease that gradually progresses to severe disability, whereas others may have one of relapse and remission. Manic depressive illness is an example of a disease, where there are *swings* from the hyperactivity associated with mania and hypomania to be followed by the depression and inactivity associated with the depressive phase.

Different outcomes and problems can arise as a consequence of the same disease. Within an individual diagnosis, such as stroke, there is considerable variation in the severity of the impairment and disability. Paralysis may be so severe that it involves the whole right side, and leaves the person incapable of speech or any other form of intellectual communication. At the other extreme, the individual may have mild impairment in speech, with difficulty in finding the occasional correct word only. It is therefore not possible, simply on the basis of a diagnostic label, to determine the consequent disability and handicap. Each individual has to be assessed as to how their disease results in specific impairment and consequent disability and handicap.

Nature of chronic disease or illness

Figure 15.3 shows the time course of the return to normal function of an individual who has suffered an acute episode of illness. (The term 'symptom threshold' is introduced at that point where an individual becomes aware that the duration or nature or severity of altered sensations merits recognition and possibly requires action.) Re-instatement of illness during remission is a relapse and during recovery is a recurrence.

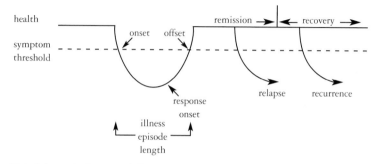

Fig. 15.3 Schematic diagram of illness episode, remission, and recovery.

Management of chronic illness

The nature, occurrence and presence of chronic diseases means that most conditions will be managed most of the time in the community. Just as the aetiology and impact are multi-factorial, so must be the management, incorporating and co-ordinating input from medical, paramedical, social, and lay bodies. The precise nature of this input will depend on the specific characteristics of the illness and the needs of the patient.

Of course, treatment should be aimed at the cause of the disease, where this is appropriate and possible (for example, avoiding allergens in asthma). However, in contrast to acute diseases, an important aim in the management of chronic diseases may be to treat the *effect*, rather than the *cause* of the disease, which might be unknown, obscure, complex, or simply untreatable. Management therefore includes minimization of impairment, control of effects, such as pain, and assistance with obtaining financial relief. The facilitation of maximal quality of life, with full realization of an individual's potential should be paramount. An important step in this management is often the change to considering a disease as chronic, rather than acute. This is sometimes difficult, requiring a potentially devastating view by the patient of him or herself. Both patient and doctor must 'admit failure' in diagnosis or cure, but the pay-off is often that profitable advances in management may be made.

SUMMARY POINTS

- In contrast to acute illness, a chronic illness often has an insidious onset, rarely has a cure, and consequently lasts for years or a lifetime.

- Modern medicines and sanitation have controlled many of the scourges of earlier days, mainly acute illnesses due to infection. The modern scourges are degenerative and chronic diseases, such as cancer and ischaemic heart disease.

- An individual's vulnerability to developing these kinds of diseases is multifactorial, i.e. it depends on an inter-play of various influences, including genetic make-up, nutrition, upbringing, and lifestyle.

- Chronic illness has effects not only on the individual, but on those around him or her, the family, and the wider community.

- The patterns that chronic disease may take are many and varied, from an acute presentation with good recovery and little persisting disability to a slow, but relentless progress with increasing disability.

- In chronic illness, in contrast to acute disease, management is mainly directed at alleviating the effects of the disease, rather than the cause (which is usually unknown or untreatable) with a view to maximizing the individual's potential and quality of life.

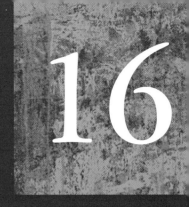

16

CHAPTER 16

Physical impairment, disability, and handicap

CHAPTER 16

Physical impairment, disability, and handicap

Introduction

This chapter provides a framework within which to consider definitions and models of disability, its epidemiology, scope for prevention, attitudes to disability, and opportunities to intervene to change its impact. This huge topic will be explored through the examples of two case histories—John and Mary.

Disability has many different implications for patients (personal, social, medical, legal, etc.), and consequences for family, friends, and community. To address this we need to develop an understanding of the resources available for the prevention of disability, and for the support and rehabilitation of those with disability in their communities.

Case histories

John

John is 33 years old and a primary school teacher. At the age of 32 he began to notice a feeling of weakness when climbing the stairs of his two-storey house, and when picking up his children aged 3 and 5. At first, he ascribed these symptoms to the pressures of work, but eventually he was persuaded to consult his GP. His GP suspected a neurological cause for his problem and John was referred to the nearest Department of Neurology, which was at the teaching hospital 45 miles away. A diagnosis of motor neuron disease was made. Over the next year, John's muscle weakness worsened and he was unable to continue with his work. Together with his family, John faces the prospect of increasing disability, and is worried about how he and his wife will cope and what resources they can draw upon.

Mary

Mary is 75 years old, living alone in a first floor flat. She has no relatives apart from a niece living in Canada. She has generalized osteoarthritis and has difficulty in fine hand movements, reaching, stretching, and climbing stairs even

> ### Mary Continued
>
> with her stick. Her right hip has become particularly stiff and painful with the result that she has stopped driving to her local supermarket and swimming club. She is now finding going out anywhere beyond the confines of her house difficult. The bus stop is 10 minutes' walk away and buses are infrequent. She finds it difficult to get on and off them. She sees her problems as one of the 'trials of old age'.

Definitions of disability

There are many different ways of defining disability. Whichever definition you are faced with, remember that disability is a descriptive term. It is not synonymous with disease or illness.

Dictionary definition

Collins Dictionary defines 'disabled' as 'lacking one or more physical powers, such as the ability to walk or to co-ordinate one's movements'. This is clear, but restricted in its outlook.

Legal definition

Criteria for disability exist in a variety of settings throughout society where rights and benefits are being considered. Doctors are often asked whether one of their patients 'qualifies' as someone with a disability. The fairness of these rules is a matter of public interest and debate and you might like to consider the role of the doctor in this exercise.

The Disability Discrimination Act (1995) defines disabled people as people who have or have had a disability that makes it difficult for them to carry out normal day-to-day activities. The disability can be physical, sensory, or mental. It must be substantial and have a long-term effect. This means the disability must last or be expected to last for 12 months.

Health definition

Medically, disability was considered within a framework published by the World Health Organization (WHO) in 1980, which is known as the International Classification of Impairments Disabilities and Handicaps (ICIDH). The definitions of impairment, disability and handicap are shown in outline (Table 16.1).

While the ICIDH provides a framework for looking at issues surrounding disability, this framework has its critics from both a philosophical and a practical point of view. Recently, to meet some of the criticisms, the WHO has conducted

Table 16.1 Definitions of impairment, disability and handicap

Pathology →	Impairment →	Disability →	Handicap
Disease Injury Congenital abnormality	Abnormalities of structure, organ or system function	Changed functional performance and activity by the individual	Disadvantage experienced by the individual as a result of impairments and disabilities
Disturbance at cellular level	Disturbance at organ level	Disturbance at personal level	Interaction at social and environmental level
Example	(1) Paralysis of limbs caused by spine bifida	(2) Having limited ability due to (1)	(3) Having fewer opportunities to work and socialize because of (2).

Source: (WHO, 1980).

trials using an updated coding system with a different nomenclature. ICIDH-2 retains the word 'impairment', but recommends that the words 'disability' and 'handicap' are no longer used. In broad terms, 'disability' becomes a restriction of *activities*, while 'handicap' becomes a reduction in participation. ICIDH-2, with its wider concepts of *impairments*, *activities*, and *participation* uses the term '*disablement*' to embrace the negative dimensions of these concepts.

Because ICIDH-2 is still being developed, throughout this chapter the 1980 terminology will be adopted.

An individual's handicaps, and his or her response to them, including the ability to participate socially, can be influenced by a wide range of factors. Some of these might include:

◆ characteristics of disability;
◆ characteristics of life before acquiring a disability;
◆ psychological factors;
◆ cultural framework;
◆ social support;
◆ social attitudes (e.g. of family, peer group, community, national);
◆ structure of environment (e.g. house, local community, workplace, etc.);
◆ economic factors;
◆ prevailing political and moral attitudes;
◆ legal framework.

In many cases when people are discussing 'disability' in a general sense outside the WHO definition, they may, in fact, be referring to the concept of 'handicap'. Think about this when listening to discussions about disability issues raised in the media and elsewhere.

Theoretical models of disability

Various perspectives on disability exist. For descriptive purposes, there has been a tendency to polarize these perspectives into two models of disability—the 'medical' model and the 'social' model. The medical model treats 'disablement' as a personal problem/ill-fortune with underlying pathological causes requiring individual intervention, often involving professionals. Management of disablement in this model is said to be aimed at promoting individual change and/or adjustment. The social model of disablement sees the issue mainly as a societal problem. Disablement is not a characteristic of a person, but a collection of conditions, many of which are created by the social environment. Management, therefore, requires social and political action to bring about change.

In the medical model, therefore, disability is said to have the following features:

- problems personal to that individual;
- requires individual treatment;
- invites professional management.

The social model features are of:

- location of the problem within society;
- individuals' limitations perceived as one factor only;
- concerns of disabled people as a group side-lined, leading to discrimination, and a need for political and social action.

Let us consider John and Mary (Table 16.2). John no longer works as a primary school teacher. Is this his 'fault' and the 'fault' of his motor neuron disease, or do his employers 'impose' disablement upon him by taking no action to enable him to teach despite his weakness?

Similarly, as far as Mary is concerned, she may have adopted a medical model of explaining her current difficulties and, indeed, medical intervention may improve her functional limitations. Might, however, her isolation and mobility difficulties be related in part to a societal problem, such as, for example, a failure of transport policy, both locally and nationally?

The medical and social models are not mutually exclusive and each has its strengths. One of the aims of the ICIDH-2 is to achieve a synthesis of these approaches. However, models of disability bring polarized views into day-to-day clinical exchanges with patients, their supporters, health and social service professionals and many others. This may lead to conflicting views on management.

Epidemiology of disability

Global perspective

The World Health Organization has estimated that over half a billion individuals (1 in 10 of the world's population) have a disability (Fig. 16.1). One-third

Table 16.2 John and Mary's disabilities

	John	Mary
Pathology	Ill-understood degeneration of motor neurons that underlies motor neuron disease	Ill-understood disorder of joints leading to osteoarthritis
Impairment	Weakness of muscles in the limbs	Limitation of joint movements, pain and stiffness
Disabilities	Difficulties in climbing stairs and picking up heavy objects (his children)	Difficulty in reaching, stretching and climbing stairs
Handicap	Given his particular impairments and disabilities, can John conduct life in the way that he wishes within his family, community and society? Can he socialize, earn a living, etc? Clearly from the details given, his circumstances have changed in at least one respect in that he is no longer teaching at the local school	Mary can no longer go to her local swimming club because of her functional difficulties. In this respect, therefore, she is disadvantaged. An interesting perspective from Mary's point of view is the social norm in relation to older people. Is it a social norm for a 75-year-old women to be driving? Some might argue (including possibly Mary herself) that her disability is 'nature's way' of telling her to give up driving. Her friends, local community and health professionals *may* also take this view

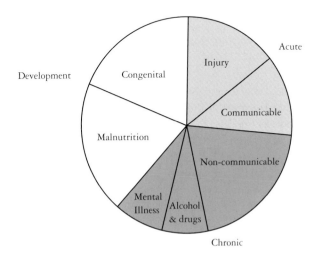

Fig. 16.1 The various classes of pathology giving rise to disability in the world.
Source: Badley & Tennant (1997).

of these are children. Over 80% of this disability is experienced by those in developing counties. Taking one specific area of disability alone, communication disability, WHO estimated in 1988 that there were 70 million individuals worldwide with hearing impairment. Recently, projections have suggested that in the developing world in 25 years' time, approximately 190 million people will have disability related to communication, which will have considerable service implications.

United Kingdom

The largest body of data we have available regarding disability in the UK stems from postal surveys and interviews done in 1985/6 and published by the Office of Population Censuses and Surveys (OPCS).

Age, sex, and severity

Figure 16.2 shows the estimates of the prevalence and severity of disability in the UK according to age and sex. You can see that both the prevalence and

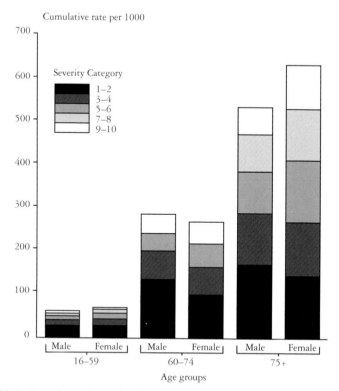

Fig. 16.2 Estimated prevalence of disability among adults by age and severity category for men and women, Great Britain, 1985–1986.
Source: OPCS (1988).

severity of disability increase with age. In the oldest age group, the proportion of women suffering from disabilities is greater than that of men. The prevalence of disability in this study among all adults was 142:1000.

Disability is not synonymous with ageing, even though Mary may think this is the case. However, it does become more common as people grow older. Over the age of 75 approximately one-third of men and half of all women report some form of disability.

Social and economic factors

Employment rates for adults with disability were shown in the OPCS Survey to be lower than those with no disability. At the time of this survey, only about one-third of disabled adults of working age were in employment. Income in this group was lower. Manual workers report more limiting problems than non-manual workers, perhaps suggesting a socio-economic group divide. Studies from the USA have also suggested ethnic differences in the prevalence of disability.

Pathology and disability

The relationship between disabilities and underlying pathologies is complex. One condition may cause several types of disability (e.g. motor neuron disease). On the other hand, a given type of disability (e.g. walking impairment) may arise from many different pathologies.

Figure 16.3 lists the main categories of disability using the OPCS surveys and the ICIDH. Figure 16.4 shows the pattern of different forms of disability based on OPCS surveys. Figure 16.4 relates to the population in Wales, but a similar graph could be constructed for Scotland, England, or Ireland. It can be seen that locomotor disability is by far the most common. Over 80% of people

OPCS	ICIDH
Locomotion	Locomotion
Personal care	Personal care
Eating, drinking & digestion	Particular skill
Reaching and stretching	Dexterity
Dexterity	Situational
Continence	Communication
Communication	Behaviour
Hearing	Sexual functioning
Seeing	Body disposition
Behaviour	
Intellectual function	
Consciousness	
Disfigurement	

Fig. 16.3 Categories of disability.

Source: OPCS (1988).

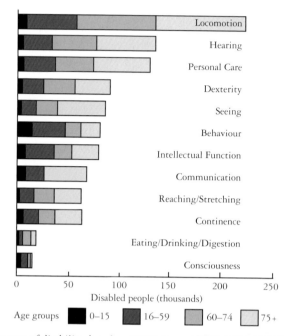

Fig. 16.4 Patterns of disability, based on OPCS Survey, 1985–1986 (OPCS, 1988).

over 75 years of age who have a disability and who live at home, have locomotor difficulties, like Mary.

Prevalence of some common pathologies

The prevalence of some common pathologies in Scotland is shown in Fig. 15.1, Chapter 15.

Mary's pathology, osteoarthritis, is top of the league table and she is likely to be one of the large number of individuals within general practice with a similar condition. Data suggest that approximately 3% of a practice population consulting in 1 year does so for osteoarthritis and the number of new cases seen by an average general practitioner per year is about 60. John's general practitioner may never see another person with newly diagnosed motor neuron disease. On average, a general practitioner sees someone with new motor neuron disease once every 33 years. John and his family will probably not know of anyone with the condition and they may feel particularly isolated because of this.

Time trends

Over the last 50 years in developed countries chronic disease, some of which has associated physical disabilities, has assumed increasing importance (see Chapter 15). In addition, an increasing proportion of the population is elderly and the relationship of increasing disability with age has been highlighted. These trends are likely to persist into the foreseeable future and have implications locally, nationally, and globally.

Attitudes to disability

A logical starting point in exploring attitudes to disability is to begin with the people you are likely to meet who have disability. Medical textbooks tend to deal with symptoms and signs, rather than the actual experiences of disability. To hear these voices you will not only have to ask those with physical disability to help you understand their experience, but seek information of this nature from the media in general, disability literature, fora and rights organizations, voluntary organizations and carers' groups, and occasionally in medical journals. Polly Toynbee, for example, wrote in *The Guardian* of the anger of her friend and fellow journalist, Jill Tweedie, at the uncomprehending and insensitive way in which health professionals dealt with disability caused by her motor neuron disease. Mary's osteoarthritis attracts little media attention, possibly because it is so common and perhaps because of its predominant occurrence in old age. Box 1 displays the attitude of one person, like Mary, who has osteoarthritis.

BOX 1

There is a tendency for strangers to assume that because you move slowly you think slowly. I have had things explained very simply and slowly for this reason, which is amusing as well as irritating. Am I angry? YES! The essential ME is lively, young, interested in all sorts of things and my body that surrounds ME is like a suit of bad-fitting armour, painful to wear and very rusty in the joints. I am annoyed that I have a complaint that can't be cured, but as long as ME is OK I feel life is good, if painful!!

The influence of language

Language has a powerful influence in shaping our attitudes towards disability, with its ability to label and isolate subgroups. There has been a historical change from using terms like 'cripple' to describe individuals with disability, to terms such as 'handicapped', 'physically challenged', 'physically impaired', 'physically different', and 'differently labelled'. There are, however, some who advocate a return to more stark terminology. The language used by people with and without disability both displays and influences their own attitudes, and those of others.

Rights for people with disability

The rights of disabled individuals are a focus of legislation, and the UK Disability Discrimination Act 1995 demands that employers and providers of services do not discriminate against people with disability. In the USA, civil rights disability legislation (Americans with Disability Act) was passed in 1990. It is difficult to evaluate the effectiveness of this legislation in improving the lives of people who have handicap.

As a provider of services, the NHS has to ensure that all people have equal access to the services they provide, both in a hospital setting and within their own communities. The challenge is for this equality of access to include all types of impairments, including John's wheelchair, Mary's stick, and people with visual and hearing impairments.

Medical responsibilities

As a health professional your attitude towards those with disabilities will have an influence in a number of areas. Negative attitudes may affect the recovery of recently disabled people. They may influence the attitude of the general public, the delivery of services, or funding decisions. You may perpetuate a negative discriminatory image by influencing further generations of students. Positive attitudes, on the other hand, may have opposite effects. Such attitudes can often be gained by listening to the many voices that have something to say about disability. This will include your patients' and their families' voices.

Cultural factors

It is recognized that different communities globally may view disabilities in different ways. Explanations for disabilities may be different, and a stigma may be attached to some disabilities and not to others. From your own cultural standpoint do you think you view different disabilities in the same way? Do you, for example, look at John differently from Mary because he is younger? It is important when considering cultural aspects of disability not to fall into stereotypes of cultural reactions and cultural myths.

Personal factors

Although this chapter deals mainly with physical disability, psychological issues are also vital. The way people respond to the onset of a disability varies enormously from person to person. Some factors that influence these psychological mechanisms are set out in Table 16.3.

Disability and the family

Disability has been discussed in individual terms and wider social terms, but within this lies the family of the person with the disability. Here, both independence

Table 16.3 Factors influencing personal reaction to disability

1. Nature of the disability	Type, severity, mode of onset, progression (including presence or absence of brain damage)
2. Information base	Knowledge, health beliefs, and expectations of person with a disability
3. Personality	Coping style, self-image, self-esteem
4. Roles	Loss, change
5. Mood	E.g. depression
6. Reaction of others	Family, friends, health professionals- and others
7. Support networks	Family, friends, local community, etc.

and interdependence are important. Thus, disability experienced by one member of the family may have far-reaching and lasting consequences for the whole family network. For John and his family there may be personal, economic, educational, and psychological repercussions for each member of the family. The perspective of other family members may differ from John's and this may lead to conflict of interest if not addressed.

Legislation was enacted in the UK in 1990 (National Health Service and Community Care Act) enabling people to live as normal a life as possible in their own homes and communities with the right amount of care and a greater say in decisions affecting their lives. Local authorities are charged with the responsibility for assessing the needs for this care, planning it, and ensuring that it is purchased and delivered appropriately. Many people with disabilities you will meet will have experienced the process of needs assessment and purchasing of care packages through local social services departments.

It has been recognized that those providing care for people with physical disabilities also need to be assessed independently. Care provided by relatives, friends, and neighbours is described officially as 'informal care'. This certainly does not mean it is uninformed care, or that it is done as an unimportant or irrelevant adjunct. Many individuals are involved in informal care in the UK. This saves the country a considerable amount of money that would otherwise need to be spent on professional care. However, there are other costs, such as the social, physical and emotional investment, the demands on time, and opportunity costs of reduced earnings. Carers need their own help and support, and a platform from which their own voices can be heard.

Disability and intervention

We need to consider the role of the general practitioner when attending an individual with impairment, disability or handicap, and his or her family. In this exercise doctors are not spectators. Identifying the pathology and impairment underlying the disability is not enough. Doctors are also concerned with the diagnosis and assessment of the disability itself, as well as in establishing its prognosis. Exploration of some of the parameters and addressing these are also important. However, intervention in disability is not the remit of the doctor alone, but of the whole multi-disciplinary health team.

Intervention to change the nature of impairments, disabilities and handicap is part of a process of rehabilitation. Box 2 shows a number of definitions of rehabilitation. They have in common the aim of maximizing an individual's potential.

BOX 2 Rehabilitation

- An active process. The restoration of patients to their fullest physical, mental, and social capability. (Scottish Home and Health Department and Scottish Health Services Council 1992)

- A process by which those disabled by injury or disease achieve a full recovery or, if full recovery is not possible, realize their optimal physical and social potential, and are integrated into their most appropriate environment. (World Health Organization 1980)

- A process of active change by which a person who has become disabled acquires and uses the knowledge and skills necessary for optimal physical, psychological, and social function. (Royal College of Physicians 1990)

- An active problem-solving and educational process, focused on disability (a person's activities) and aiming to maximize the patient's participation in society and his or her well-being while reducing stress on the family. This includes assessment (diagnosis of the underlying impairments and disorders), the setting of goals, and provision of care to maintain the patient's state. (Wade 1999)

Two approaches to intervention in disability have been described, echoing the medical and social models of disability, respectively. There is a therapeutic approach and a prosthetic approach. In the therapeutic model, intervention is aimed at changing the nature of the disability. So, for example, in Mary's case surgical replacement of her right hip joint may lessen her disability, and alter her need for services and aids and appliances around and about the house. In the prosthetic approach, the environment is adapted by various means to allow the person with the disability to go about their wished everyday activities of life. Ramps providing access to buildings for people in wheelchairs are an example of this. In reality, rehabilitation adopts both therapeutic and prosthetic approaches in day-to-day clinical practice.

The effectiveness of rehabilitation in producing health and social gain is a matter of considerable debate and research. There is good evidence that it can change outcomes for people who have had strokes, and there is promising evidence in other fields such as following hip fractures and acquired brain injury, heart attacks and coronary artery surgery. Interventions can also be targeted at individual impairments and disabilities such as treatments for incontinence and visual and hearing impairments.

There may be considerable cost implications of new interventions that may have an impact on impairments and disability. These include newer and expensive treatments such as cochlear implantation for children with hearing impairment, beta interferon for multiple sclerosis, Riluzole© for slowing the course of motor neuron disease (which John may wish), sildenafil (Viagra©) for impotence, botulinum toxin for spasticity, etc. It is important that new interventions are thoroughly evaluated for effectiveness and safety before their routine use in the NHS. However, media and public pressure often demands their use before evaluation is completed.

Practical issues in rehabilitation

Rehabilitation is a multidisciplinary endeavour. Figures 16.5 and 16.6 indicate the kind of input that might be offered to John and his family. Knowledge of

- ◆ General practitioner
- ◆ Physiotherapy—maintenance of mobility fitness, etc.
- ◆ Occupational Therapy—assessment of activities of daily living, provision of aids and appliances, adaptations to environment, vocational aspects, therapeutic interventions, etc.
- ◆ District Nurses—help with bowel care, treatment of any pressure areas, etc.
- ◆ Dieticians
- ◆ Speech and Language Therapy—communication issues, swallowing difficulties
- ◆ Social Services (e.g. social worker)
  - Provision of rights and benefits
  - Contact with other appropriate agencies
  - Access to day centres
  - Respite care
  - Support for the family
  - Night and day sitter services
- ◆ Other Services in the Community
  - Housing
  - Department of Employment
  - Leisure
  - Church
  - Educational support for children
  - Local self help groups and disability fora

Fig. 16.5 Community resources.

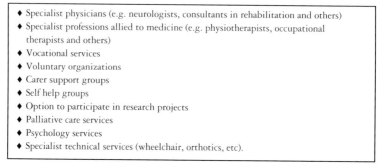

♦ Specialist physicians (e.g. neurologists, consultants in rehabilitation and others)
♦ Specialist professions allied to medicine (e.g. physiotherapists, occupational therapists and others)
♦ Vocational services
♦ Voluntary organizations
♦ Carer support groups
♦ Self help groups
♦ Option to participate in research projects
♦ Palliative care services
♦ Psychology services
♦ Specialist technical services (wheelchair, orthotics, etc).

Fig. 16.6 Resources beyond the immediate general practice/community.

the existence of local and national resources is important in order to activate these. It is also important that this input is driven by and tailored to the needs of John and his family, and is co-ordinated and confidential.

Reflect on the number of professionals and others who can potentially become involved in John's household. What will be the impact of this parade of people on John and his family's life? Is it unacceptably intrusive and what will be its impact in terms of his control over his own situation? Who should co-ordinate it—should it be John? Will everyone's roles be clearly understood? What are the implications for health resources? Is the picture different for Mary?

Conclusions

Disability is a complex and topical issue. Health professionals are faced with people presenting with a wide range of disabilities in their practices, seeking advice and help. No two handicaps are the same and each person will want to agree a tailored programme to meet their particular goals. The 1995 Disability Discrimination Act may focus all our minds on the extent to which we discriminate against individuals with disability in providing services. People with disability are demanding a central say in how health services are planned and delivered, and that they are given proper choice and information. John and Mary need informed doctors in all these important areas.

SUMMARY POINTS

♦ Disability can be defined in different ways. The dictionary definitions, legal definition, and WHO's definitions have different implications. Disability is not synonymous with disease or illness.

SUMMARY POINTS Continued

◆ In the health (WHO) context, an individual's difficulties can be mediated by a wide range of factors, including the characteristics of the disability, what his or her life was like beforehand, psychological, social, cultural, environmental and economic factors, prevailing political and moral attitudes, and the legal framework.

◆ For descriptive purposes only (though these are not 'real' divisions) there is a 'medical' and a 'social' way of looking at disability, with corresponding implications, but these are not mutually exclusive approaches. The best approach is a synthesis of the two.

◆ Worldwide, 1 in 10 individuals has a disability and a third of all of these are children. Most people with disabilities (80%) live in developing countries. Disability increases with age. In the UK one-third of men and half of women over 75 years of age report some form of disability, locomotor disability being by far the most common.

◆ Positive legislation (such as in UK and USA) can help prevent unwitting discrimination against people with disabilities, e.g. in providing equality of access.

◆ Health professionals must carefully examine their own attitudes to disability lest they perpetuate negative discriminating attitudes by influencing further generations of students. Positive attitudes have positive effects.

◆ Intervention in disability is part of the process of rehabilitation and is a team, rather than an individual, activity.

References and further reading

For recent publications relating to the World Health Organization International Classification of Functioning, Disability and Health (ICIDH-2), consult the ICIDH website: http://www.who.int/icidh/

Badley & Tennant (1997). Epidemiology, in Goodwill, C.J., Chamberlain, M.A., Evans, C. (eds.), *Rehabilitation of the Physically Disabled Adult*. Stanley Thornes Ltd, Cheltenham.

Edwards, F.C. & Warren, M.D. (1990). *Health Services for Adults with Physical Disabilities*. Royal College of Physicians: London.

Goodwill, C.J. & Chamberlain, M.A. (Eds) (1988). *Rehabilitation of the Physically Disabled Adult*. Croom Helm, London.

OPCS (1988). *The Prevalence of Disability Among Adults*. OPCS, London.

Patrick, D.L. & Peach, H. (1998). *Disablement in the Community*. Oxford University Press, Oxford.

Scottish Home and Health Department and Scottish Health Services Council (1992). *Medical Rehabilitation: the Pattern for the Future*. HMSO, Edinburgh.

Swain, J., Finkelstein, V., French, S. & Oliver, M. (Eds) (1992). *Disabling Barriers—Enabling Environments*. Open University Press, Buckingham/SAGE, London.

Wade, D. (1999). Rehabilitation therapy after stroke. *Lancet*, **354**, 176–7.

World Health Organization (1980). *International Classification of Impairments, Disabilities and Handicaps*. WHO, Geneva.

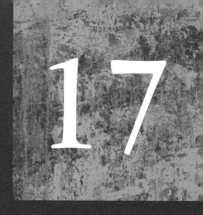

CHAPTER 17

Psychological problems in the community

CHAPTER 17

Psychological problems in the community

Psychological vulnerability

The risk of mental symptoms is not distributed evenly in the population. Some individuals for reason of their circumstances, their occupation, or their family antecedents are at greater risk of becoming mentally ill than others. Psychological factors also make slight, but consistent contributions to the risk of some types of physical illness, such as heart disease. These factors may be developmental (e.g. learning difficulties, personality, and ageing) or environmental (e.g. marital stress and occupation). We need to be aware of how extensive mental health issues are in healthcare in the community and how an integrative approach to psychological, social, and biological determinants of mental well-being can be rewarding for both patient and doctor.

The child or young adult with learning difficulties

BOX 1 Causes of learning difficulty

Children and adults with learning difficulties are categorized throughout history under numerous headings, such as imbecile, idiot, mental retardation, or mental handicap. Contemporary use of the term 'learning difficulty' avoids some of the stigmatization of the past. Causes of learning difficulties are broadly grouped into genetic, acquired, mixed, and unknown. Known causes (e.g. chromosomal anomaly) account for a greater proportion of severe degree of learning difficulties than moderate to mild.

The child or young adult with learning difficulties (Box 1) is at greater risk of mental disorder than their non-impaired counterparts. The greater risk extends to physical disease and higher mortality. These associations probably derive from less efficient use of health services, acquisition of behaviours hazardous to health (smoking and poor diet) and social processes. These last are unclear in their precise mechanisms, but are likely to be closely linked to social setting or family group. Mild to moderate degrees of learning difficulty arise more often in families exposed to socio-economic hardships. These families may suffer the multiple handicaps of poor nutrition, overcrowding, unemployment, alcohol and substance abuse, and possibly inherited causes of learning difficulty. The term 'intergenerational cycles of disadvantage' was coined to describe families affected in this way.

Insight and learning difficulty

Examination of the child or young adult with learning difficulties provides useful lessons in understanding the nature and importance to mental health of particular types of judgement and reasoning. Social learning in childhood and adolescence is accompanied by the acquisition and later refinement of 'insight'. This term is difficult to define with precision. In clinical medicine, it is used to describe the understanding of a patient about the nature of their illness. This has obvious implications for the extent with which that patient might comply with or consent to treatment of the illness. It also has implications for the patient's understanding of the future impact of this illness on their lifestyle.

Insight is used in psychology and psychiatry in a second quite distinct way. Here, 'insight' can be used to describe the ability to develop within one's own mind a mental model of a problem (Box 2). This is important when trying to address a problem such as illness. People with learning difficulties tend to have less insight and, therefore, to have more problems with illness.

BOX 2 Mental imagery in chimpanzees

The best known example of this form of reasoning derives from laboratory observations on chimpanzees about 75 years ago. The laboratory area contained apparently random objects (sticks, rope, boxes) scattered around. Faced with a bunch of bananas placed above their reach a chimp will jump unsuccessfully or attempt to dislodge a banana with a thrown stick until retiring apparently to rest. After an interval, some chimps will pick up boxes in the laboratory, place one on the other, climb to the top, and take the fruit. The inference is made that the chimp has 'solved' the problem by reflecting on the problem, constructing a mental image of the issues involved, and acting to effect the solution.

Learning difficulties and social attachment

The environment provides important resources to assist the individual to cope adequately with adversity. Resilience of this variety largely derives from the emotional bonds formed by a child first with parents and then outside the family. Most children with learning difficulties establish these social bonds more slowly, there are fewer of them and they are less effective than in non-learning disabled children. This sort of delayed or uneven social development is the proper focus of most community-based special education provisions made for children with learning difficulties. Their inability to make insightful judgements about relationships, especially with potentially exploitative adults, determines their needs for some form of protection often well into adult life. This is part of the duty of a responsible society to care for vulnerable people. When social networks are ineffective, resources available to overcome adversity to the child or young adult with learning difficulties are limited. Consequently, emotional reactions to distress may threaten to overwhelm the youngster leading to protracted unwanted behaviour patterns. These can be very difficult to contain or modify, and are best prevented; optimum management requires review of social development and the establishment of lasting affectionate relationships. Family and community are therefore of vital importance in managing learning difficulties.

Failure to learn social lessons is also accompanied by limited skills in the use of language. This limitation restricts the learning disabled child's ability to describe changes in internal feelings. Inappropriate explanations may be offered to describe mental life. In the absence of a useful range of vocabulary to reflect thoughts and feelings, the child may complain about mental problems (like the sadness of depression) in physical terms such as 'headache' or 'tummy pain'. Difficulties with the correct use of language and misunderstanding relationships between what is self and non-self can severely impair the child's assessment of what is happening, especially when events are potentially stressful or ambiguous. In normal healthy childhood, magical beliefs, rigid morality, and impulsivity are commonplace and appropriate from age 3 to 7 years. In the learning disabled child this manner of thinking can persist into adulthood. Even with special care, modification of these features (appropriate to early childhood development) is not so readily established. Social, cognitive, and emotional development is usually slower and less well integrated in the presence of learning difficulties. Severe mental illnesses are about 10 times more frequent in adults with mild to moderate forms of learning difficulty. When these syndromes are also linked to the presence of epilepsy and/or clear evidence of neuro-developmental abnormality, assessment, and optimum management are difficult.

Personality problems in adults

The term personality is used to describe those traits or characteristics which define an individual's uniqueness (see also Chapter 10). Methods to detect and measure personality and its disorders are of three broad types: categorical, developmental, and dimensional. Used alone, none of these methods is entirely satisfactory in clinical practice. The categorical approach to personality and its disorders rests on the assumption that the majority of individuals conform to a 'normal' stereotype, and that there are several groups of outliers each with typical features. Clinical interests in the outliers rests on the idea that these individuals are more vulnerable to the development of mental illness than the 'normal' type. For example, one group is more likely to break the law, use illicit substances, and show a callous disregard for the feelings of others. An older typology uses the term 'psychopath' to denote this particular constellation of traits. Traits are relatively enduring, usually established by adolescence and quite distinct from states that are transient. Another category of personality disorder shows lack of interest in social involvement, preference for solitary pursuits, abstract thinking and poor motivation. For this, the terms 'schizotypy' or 'schizoid' were introduced. The clinical interest here was the possibility that individuals with these types of personality were more likely to become schizophrenic than others. Likewise, terms like 'obsessional personality' were linked to later development of obsessive compulsive disorder, and 'pyknic' types or 'cyclothymic personalities' were believed more likely to develop manic depressive disorder. The importance of these notions is that they contain two features. First, each of the categories of personality is a composite of a large number of traits that may be present to a greater or lesser extent, and secondly, they may also be continuous with 'normal personality'. These two ideas led to the dimensional theory of personality that rests on responses to paper and pencil personality questionnaires. To be properly comprehensive, personality questionnaires must contain sufficient items to identify the wide range of traits, attitudes, and behaviours, which are believed to distinguish between personality types (see also Types A and B personality in Chapter 10).

The older person

In growing old, friendships depleted by death and failing physical health pose important problems for some old people. When the resources available to overcome stressful events are depleted, the risk of mental disorder is increased. Obvious psychological changes with ageing are linked to retirement from work. This is not sudden, for productivity may decline from about age 40. There may be reduced energy, motivation, and often increased interests outside work. There are also age-related declines in mental speed and intelligence, partly compensated for by acquisition and consolidation of other mental skills and problem-solving abilities.

Psychological ageing begins around age 50 and is well established by age 75. Social ageing is affected by life-long patterns of social adjustment. Maintenance of mental effort, certain features of character and temperament, and interest in the meaning of personal experience all define an individual's self-perception in old age.

Social adjustment in old age is often represented by processes of disengagement when old people gradually withdraw from society. Friends may die, children move away, travelling may require much effort, and there may be fears of falls. Although disengagement seems a sensible strategy, it is fraught with hazard. Without a social network to support and advise, the older person is at risk of development of symptoms of mental disorder.

Some mental symptoms are linked with ageing. These include the pervasive sense of despair ('demoralization'), which often affects older people as they struggle to manage their emotions in the face of bereavement or other losses. These include not just the loss of people, but of self-esteem (linked to social rank), skills, and sensory ability. As concentration powers are impaired by mental symptoms (like anxiety and depression), so the older person may worry about the symptoms of early dementia.

BOX 3 Old age

Changes in sensory abilities are among the clearest mental changes with ageing. Hearing loss is the best studied. From age about 32 in men and 37 in women, people complain about their hearing. Perception of higher frequencies (in the 4000–6000 Hz range, but most marked over 8000 Hz) is reduced. Hearing loss of this form is very common and impairs not just conversation, but the ability to make new friends. Visual senses are also impaired by ageing. The basic principles of brain plasticity were first worked out for the visual cortex. With ageing, the same brain plastic processes compensate for visual impairment. The best known example is the slow formation of cataracts in the lens of the eye that begins around age 20. As the cataract forms, the ageing brain adjusts to the changed properties of the image relayed from the retina. One of the most remarkable experiences for an older person is to have visual acuity restored by a replacement lens.

Visual and auditory misperceptions with ageing may predispose isolated, anxious older people to become suspicious about their world. In some susceptible, vulnerable individuals these suspicions come to dominate their thinking. Intense beliefs of a persecutory nature are termed 'paranoid' and may become delusions. (Delusions are false beliefs that are held with certainty and are not explained by the individual's cultural or religious convictions.)

Change in the social integration of older people in society poses a considerable and chronic stress. They may feel less involved and less valued by the society they helped to create. Some older people say they feel alienated from a society so preoccupied by health, youth, beauty, and the display of material wealth. Previously, close and frequent ties within an extended family and within a small local community helped maintain mental well-being. Now, families are smaller and social activities much more age-stratified than before. Attitudes to older people are sometimes negative, which may reinforce a sense of social rejection or exclusion.

The physically handicapped child or young adult

The impact of physical handicap on the individual depends on the nature and extent of the handicap, and degree of central nervous system involvement. Self-esteem, body image, personal attractiveness, mobility, and family reactions to the physical handicap are each powerful determinants of the vulnerability of the physically handicapped individual to mental symptoms.

Dependency on others is most often entirely outside the handicapped person's control. Reactions include withdrawal from relationships and unhappiness. When parents react in an extreme fashion (over-protectiveness or excessive criticism) a handicapped child's anger at first may seem unreasonable and tantrum-like. Sometimes, however, this is the only option open to the child whose parents allow him or her little or no personal say.

Early sexual development is compromised by the handicapped child's reliance on others for assistance with personal hygiene. A sense of modesty and privacy develops in normal childhood, but this is delayed when a child is handicapped. The intimacy of personal contact between parent and child, when it persists into adolescence, may even hinder private discussions about sexual matters so that the handicapped individual remains emotionally less mature and resilient than their peers.

Long-term relationships under stress

Studies of the causes of mental disorders like alcoholism, suicide, anxiety, and depression, point to marital stress as an important factor. Most classical studies have been of the husband/wife relationship within marriage, but they may well apply to other long-term relationships, whether of different or the same sexes. The association is not well understood, but several features of relationships under stress are consistently linked with mental symptoms. The first problem about the relationship concerns the people involved. Were they always like this? Did the relationship do this to them? Did he/she make him/her like this? The choice of partner is of obvious relevance. Do people with mental symptoms (or a predisposition to develop symptoms) tend to form long-term relationships with one another? This is called 'assortative mating' in which like chooses like. There is no good evidence that this is the case, but it is true that a person who marries someone with minor mental symptoms will become more like that person as they remain together.

If assortative mating does not take place, what about processes within the relationship, which may influence the 'well' partner? The 'sick' person is known to demand much more contact with their 'well' partner than is usual in symptom-free, unstressed couples. Potentially, the influence of the 'sick' over the 'well' partner could derive from hidden (latent) traits in the 'well' partner being uncovered or activated by the 'sick' partner. If it is assumed in life that there are two important sets of intimate relationships (the first with one's parents and the second with one's own long-term partner) then patterns of behaviour established in childhood (including the acquisition of specific defence mechanisms) may be re-activated in a long-term partnership. These may lead to loss of self-esteem, a sense of rejection, and hostility. In such terms the 'sick' person chooses a mate with some of the characteristics of one or both their parents. Within the relationship, the 'sick' partner re-establishes an approximation to the relationship within their original family. Their relationship with the 'well' partner leads to this person using 'defence mechanisms' excessively to preserve the integrity of the sense of self or separateness. This is a commonplace explanation of the processes that lead to married couples becoming more alike in the expression of mental symptoms and personal maladjustment. It also provides an explanation for some types of breakdown of long-term relationships.

A long-term relationship is usually continuous and excludes others. In terms of attachment theory (see Chapter 10), anxiety, and depression are experienced when exclusivity of the bond is endangered. The bond will be threatened if one partner resists the processes described above. Affective reactions to the real or imagined breakdown of the relationship are widespread. They are modified by the stage of development of the relationship. In the early years, withdrawal from parents, family, and friends may cause problems especially when one of the partners does not negotiate the process. Here, one or several relationships are allowed to take precedence over the relationship with the partner (e.g. with mother or a previous close friend).

BOX 4 Sex

Sexual relationships are subject to the competing pressures of work or unemployment. They are affected by tiredness, time away from home, and the care taken to be a considerate lover. Children introduce a layer of complexity for which the relationship may be unprepared. Although joy is universally linked

> **BOX 4** Continued
>
> with the birth of a child, the father may feel subsequently excluded from the mother's intense new relationship. This sense of exclusion is made greater if (as is common) the mother suffers from a depressive illness after childbirth. Relationships with one's parents re-emerge during this phase of marriage as important determinants of feelings towards the partner. If these were unsatisfactory, either partner may anticipate rejection and feel unwanted. In reaction, their dependent need to hold onto the female partner may cause a male partner to become clinging, intrusive, and hostile.

People under stress at work

Job selection is not simply a matter of matching ability to do the job with the motivation and wage rewards. Job satisfaction rates highly for many as does the morale and a sense of personal development linked to some types of work. Some jobs are thought stressful and sometimes also pay well. Extra earnings are not linked directly to the stressful nature of work, but more often to the health hazards associated with this sort of work. The stressful nature of the work may serve to attract some individuals to do the job. Explanations vary between workers but, when asked, some say the work is exciting because it is stressful, others that it is more worthwhile (to the public good) or that this kind of work will make them a better person. Military recruitment exploits this type of motivation with slogans such as 'We'll make a man of you!' implying that with proper training and involvement with crises, selected individuals will return to society 'steeled' by the experience of stress. This is true not just of military personnel but of emergency services, health workers, and even some categories of child care; the list is very long.

The promotion of personal growth is an objective of many management development programmes. Some include simulations of military training with games designed to test or stress participants. Lessons learnt here are expected to be transferred to the workplace, where the worker trained in this way is expected to require less external direction and to use more self-control. The employee who is trained to use stress at work in this formative way will gain new rewards in terms of improved morale and better motivation. Failure to achieve this degree of personal development is linked to inefficient or rigid working practices (to avoid exposure to stress at work), and the abuse of alcohol or drugs.

Other medical conditions are linked to failure to manage stress at work. These are decreased consultation threshold to seek medical care and time off work, cardiovascular disorders, hypertension, stroke, myocardial infarction, sudden death (often unexplained), and accidents. The physiological mechanisms that link stress at work to disease (especially cardiovascular disease) are not well understood. The first ideas suggest that these types of complication are more properly linked to socio-economic deprivation. People who have poorly paid jobs can only afford poor housing in neighbourhoods with high overcrowding, unemployment, and chronic fear of theft or violence. Their culture does not resist pressures to smoke or drink. Low pay determines a need to work long hours and to rely on public transport. Time available for shopping and recreation is less, and so convenience or cheaper high calorific foods become an important part of the diet. Sometimes, when alcohol is taken it may be intended to have a rapid effect. As much as can be afforded is taken as quickly as possible. In these circumstances workers have little opportunity to escape from living conditions that predispose to ill health. They are exposed to new risks of disease and substance abuse.

The second idea focuses much more on the work itself. This is supported by studies of the chances of dying among otherwise similar groups of workers. In a large prospective study of Bell telephone employees those who worked full time and also attended evening classes were more likely to die of myocardial infarction than those who were similar in other respects, but did not 'overwork' in this way. Likewise individuals in large corporations who feel they work 'under severe pressure' are more likely 10 years later to be dead than those who do not self-report in this way. Other studies have shown that the risk of premature death is linked to changes in work practices (changes from a nationalized to a commercial bank, for example) and group pressures to maintain piece work rates. These types of study show that the nature of work and how it is managed determine its impact on the individual with important consequences for health. It is certain that ageing, work pattern, income inequalities and work strain are linked in a complex way to determine risks to mental and physical health.

Shift work

Just as there are temporal rhythms in physiological processes, so psychological functions display marked time of day effects. The term 'circadian' was introduced to describe the usual period of daily rhythms, i.e. each lasted about a day's length (around 25 hours). In the absence of environmental time cues to 'reset' or entrain these rhythms, they tend to 'free run' moving out of step with the day length by a fixed time difference with each cycle. The physiological control of internal time keeping (the biological clock) is provided by a paired system of brain nuclei each oscillating at different frequencies and together capable of generating rhythms that vary in length from infradian (around 90 min) to circadian (around 25 h) to ultradian, which may be monthly, seasonal or annual.

The purpose of integrated rhythmicity in physiological and psychological functions in complex nervous systems is poorly understood. The underlying principles probably include the need to anticipate regular environmental change and so make optimum use of environmental opportunities to compete for food and raise young.

BOX 5 Jet lag and shift work

When entrainment with the environment is artificially desynchronized the individual suffers important consequences with implications for the maintenance of health. Rapid transmeridian travel across several time zones often produces transient physical and psychological symptoms. These phenomena are well known as 'jet lag'. Similarly, there are the health problems of shift workers subject to regular rotas of shift duty which demand periods of adjustment to work patterns that may be 4, 8 or 12 hours out of synchrony with the more usual day shift (08.00–17.00 hours). Health studies of shift workers reveal excess complaints of back pain, sleep disturbance, low mood, more frequent accidents, and greater absenteeism. This excess is probably due to the failure of some individuals to adapt successfully to shift working.

Desynchronization in shift work leads to a decrease in overall psychological performance efficiency. Decreased vigilance probably explains the excess of accidents during night shifts. Fortunately, only about 5% of the work force follows fixed work shift patterns with night alternating with day shifts and rest periods. A further 35% work irregular hours. Careful attention to the construction of shift work rotas can reduce the disruptive effects of shift work, and improve absenteeism and health of shift workers.

Is work stressful?

Hectic work patterns, excessive overtime, and conflict between work and family responsibilities differ between individuals in terms of their harmful effects. Some report more satisfaction, while others feel constantly under strain. It is not unusual for workers in this position to develop negative views about their work, their managers, and some of their colleagues. These views are typically expressed with sarcasm or cynicism, workers may belittle junior or less assertive colleagues, and this is one form of bullying at work. Finally, the victims of bullying may develop mental symptoms of sufficient severity to impair their capacity to work.

SUMMARY POINTS

◆ Psychological factors may promote mental and physical disorders in any of us, but some groups of individuals are particularly vulnerable.

◆ This chapter discusses the particular problems of children and young adults with learning difficulties and physical handicap.

SUMMARY POINTS Continued

◆ It also discusses how some individuals may be especially vulnerable to the stresses of ageing, marriage, and work, and how vulnerability may relate to personality.

◆ Finally, there is an explanation of how psychological vulnerability may arise from the conflicting demands of work and personal life, concluding with the specific example of the stressful biological effects of shift working.

References and further reading

Porter, M., Alder, B. & Abraham, C. (1999). *Psychology and Sociology Applied to Medicine: an illustrated colour text.* Churchill Livingston, Edinburgh.

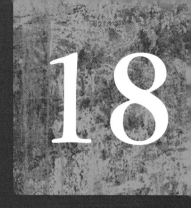

CHAPTER 18
Death and dying

CHAPTER 18
Death and dying

Death: natural process or failure of medicine

There is a time to be born and a time to die. (Ecclesiastes 3, v2)

Dying is part of our human experience. Death is one of the great mysteries of life. For many there is faith in a spiritual life beyond the grave, but from the moment of birth we begin on our physical journey of life that will end in death for each one of us. We live in community, touched by the life and death of others:

No man is an Iland, intire of it selfe; . . .
any man's death diminishes me, because I am involved in Mankinde;
and therefore never send to know for whom the bell tolls;
it tolls for thee.

(John Donne, 1572–1631)

Yet in our post-modern society death is so often hidden in institutions and seldom acknowledged. In the Middle Ages, when mortality rates were high and open to marked fluctuations, death was viewed as familiar and commonplace, an inevitable and public event. Places of burial were also public places in the community used for markets and judicial proceedings. Christianity was the dominant religious belief in Britain and importance laid on preparation for meeting with God. Over the next centuries focus in the church doctrine moved to the last judgement. Art and literature focused on the need to 'die well'. *Ars Morendi*, 'the art of dying' for example, is a fascinating account of how to prepare for death. In the nineteenth century, rituals around death moved to those bereaved. Death became romanticized and mourning, not dying, the central act.

Medicine

The Hippocratic tradition was to not treat those deemed to be incurable. The doctor should not challenge nature and, therefore, the gods, lest he pay the penalty for his presumption. This view was tempered with changes in culture and religion, but even in the nineteenth century, a physician had far fewer therapeutic options available compared to his modern colleagues. In the last stages of life his role was to be alongside the patient keeping vigil and alleviating suffering. His professional presence was needed to mark the change from life to death, but less often to prevent it. In the words of a sixteenth century aphorism:

A physician's role is
to cure sometimes,
to relieve often
to comfort always.

In the twentieth century with changes in culture, religion, public health, and medical advances, death became seen as the enemy of the doctor. No longer was it the clergy wrestling with the one dying to prepare for an afterlife, but rather the doctor actively intervening to prevent early and premature death. Along with the reduction in infant and maternal mortalities, the change in the pattern of mortality, increased life expectancy, and developments in modern medicine, death became removed from the community. Although most of the last year of life is still spent at home, death commonly occurs in an institutional setting and within a medical context. Many adults will never have seen a relative die and may not experience a close bereavement until their 30s or later. Although the twentieth century saw an unparalleled increase in human-induced and violent death, such as the concentration camps, world wars, and atomic bombs, doctors practise in a death-denying culture. Death is the modern taboo.

Over the past 100 years we have witnessed what is popularly called the 'miracle of modern medicine'. Undreamed of advances in technology have brought the antibiotic era, anaesthetics and anti-sepsis allowing dramatic surgical advances, radiology, radiotherapy and chemotherapy, immunology, endocrinology, gene therapy, and organ transplantation. Doctors have become primarily diagnosticians and therapists, hospitals places of investigation, treatment, and discharge, and death is, at best, a medical failure and, at worst, a statistical embarrassment. Popular expectation is that there are no boundaries to the life-saving scope of medical knowledge and technology. Perhaps in the twenty-first century we are beginning to see a change in this attitude. There is a fear that life must be prolonged at all costs regardless of its quality.

When and why do people die?

The past 150 years have seen a marked change in the patterns of mortality, along with other substantial changes in the population relating to demography and levels of health. In the 1850s perinatal mortality was high—more than 150 deaths per 1000 live births in England and Wales. Maternal death rates were high often due to puerperal infection and did not decline until the 1930s.

Infectious diseases accounted for 1 in 3 deaths in the mid-nineteenth century with the highest individual cause being tuberculosis. The influenza pandemic of 1918–19 resulted in 21 million deaths—more than twice the number of combat deaths in World War 1.

The two most common causes of death today are cancer and ischaemic heart disease (see Chapter 3). These two causes each accounted for almost a quarter of all deaths in Scotland in 1998. Since 1995 there have been more deaths from cancer than from ischaemic heart disease. Causes of death vary with different age groups. In the young (aged 1–14), accidents account for 38% of deaths in boys and 23% in girls. In men aged 15–34, suicide is the main cause. For the main cause of death, cancer, there are trends in terms of overall rates, specific sites, and disease trajectory. These figures vary within the UK, e.g. Glasgow had the highest standardized ratio for cancer of the lung, 52% higher than the Scottish average. When deaths due to diseases of the circulatory system are grouped together they account for 43% of all deaths and continue to show a gradual decline.

In 1995 the life expectancy in England and Wales was 74.4 years compared with less than 40 years in the mid-1800s. For Scots, life expectancy has also increased—since 1861 by 32.3 years for men and 34.1 years for women. At birth a Scotsman in 1998 could expect a span of 72.6 years and a Scotswoman 78.1 years. Figure 18.1 shows average age at death for Scotland. Note the troughs caused by the World Wars and the influenza pandemic.

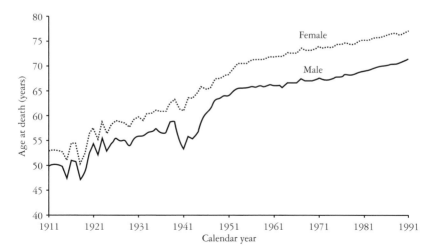

Fig. 18.1 Average age at death in Scotland.

When death is unexpected

Unexpected 'natural' or traumatic death

Unexpected death, particularly when the circumstances are traumatic, causes a profound sense of shock. This may be further compounded by the associated legal requirements. There is no opportunity to say goodbye, to resolve differences or to take back those last hasty words. For some there is a sense of relief caused by the sudden nature of the loss: 'at least he didn't suffer'. The professionals involved may not know the patient or family, particularly if the death occurs in hospital. Continuity of care may therefore be a problem, so good communication with the primary care team is essential.

Multiple deaths from road traffic accidents or other disasters/violence

The overwhelming nature of these types of loss make adjustment more difficult. There may be multiple deaths and nobody to help assert the reality. This is compounded by the involvement of the police, Coroner, or Procurator Fiscal with subsequent legal proceedings and a climate of blame. The bereaved person may have been involved in the tragedy or be overwhelmed by the trauma. Their experience may be further swamped by media attention. Think of events such as the Piper Alpha oil rig explosion in the North Sea in 1988 when 167 men died, or the Kings Cross fire in the London Underground station in 1987 when 32 people died.

Unexpected deaths of children

Perhaps more than any other these events carry a sense of shock, helplessness, and blame. The death of a child strikes at the heart of our shared future. There is the loss of the vulnerable individual along with all the potential that child represented.

Sudden infant death syndrome (or cot death) has the difficulty of no definite diagnosis and may carry the stigma of parental blame. Coping with the loss of an adolescent may also be particularly difficult because relationships may be ambivalent, and the cause of death is more likely to be accident or suicide. The following quotes are from parents of teenagers killed at the Hillsborough disaster in 1989 when 96 Liverpool football supporters died from crush injuries:

◆ there is this enormous feeling of inadequacy. The time they need you most. What can you do?
◆ shock, I suppose. I had never, never, experienced anything like that in my life. This feeling of unreality, this dreamlike state.
◆ it's almost like being inside your own little time capsule ... You're working on autopilot.

Professionals involved, such as police officers, paramedics, accident and emergency staff, chaplains, social workers, and the general practitioner, can find it difficult to cope with their own sense of outrage and powerlessness. One of the ambulance drivers who attended the Dunblane School in Scotland, where 16 children and their teacher were killed in a gun massacre in March 1996, said:

> I can only describe what I saw as a medieval vision of hell.

A message left outside the school read:

> May God take better care of you than this world ever did.

A tragedy like this affects a wider community. Helen Liddell, MP said:

> This is a slaughter of the innocents, unlike anything we have ever seen in Scotland, and I think Scotland is going to have to come to terms with it.

This tragedy led directly to legislation abolishing the possession of handguns in the UK.

When death is expected

Definitions

Terminal care is the last phase of care when a patient's condition is deteriorating and death is close. Terminal illness is an emotive and misleading term that is usually only applied to cancer from the time of diagnoses. There is the implication of dying, rather than living throughout the illness. There may be a worse prognosis with other conditions, e.g. after a myocardial infarction and left ventricular damage. Palliative care is, therefore, a more helpful term for the management of illnesses such as cancer, until the terminal phase is reached.

Palliative care/symptom management

Palliative care is a philosophy of care that emphasizes quality of life. The focus is on symptom control, integrating the psychological and spiritual aspects of care, and offering support to families both during the patient's illness and in their bereavement. This approach to care should be offered by a multidisciplinary team and in many ways enshrines good medical care for any chronic illness. Most palliative care is provided by the primary health care team, with support from specialist practitioners and specialist palliative care units (or hospices).

Pain is the symptom most feared by patients with cancer, but is also common in the terminal stages of many illnesses. However, no symptom (including pain) should be addressed in isolation and all symptoms affect each other. Anxiety, for example, increases pain, and vice-versa. It is important, therefore, in planning palliative care, to begin by listening carefully and completely to the patient's experiences and needs, and to respond globally. Palliative care is a dynamic process that will need to change its focus as the disease and the experience of it progress. It is important throughout to set goals that are both realistic and shared by all concerned.

CASE STUDY 1

Fiona is a 35-year-old woman with advanced colorectal cancer that was diagnosed 2 months ago after a delay in diagnosis. She is currently receiving chemotherapy. She has pain due to liver secondaries, and finds the morphine painkillers make her nauseated and drowsy. You adjust her analgesia to control her pain without unacceptable side effects in discussion with the Palliative Medicine Consultant.

However, you talk further and discover she is a single mother with three children, the youngest of whom, Sam, is 5 years old. There has been no discussion as to the future of the children and she is struggling to find childcare when she is in hospital. She has no contact with the children's father and does not want him to have custody. The oldest child, Becky, is 11 years old and is asking a lot of questions her mother does not know how to answer.

You involve other members of the team, namely the social worker and Macmillan nurse. You begin to talk about her poor prognosis. As her disease and symptoms progress her chemotherapy is discontinued, and you arrange for an admission to the specialist palliative care unit for symptom control. She deteriorates quickly and is now dying. However, she is very distressed and asks to see the chaplain. She is frightened and agitated. As the chaplain explores her fears Fiona says she had always planned to be baptized in her local church, but kept putting it off. She now knows she is dying and wants a service in the unit. With her family present Fiona is baptized by the chaplain and dies peacefully a few hours later.

Communication/psychological care

Good communication is essential to good palliative care. Poor communication is one of the most common causes of distress reported by patients and their families. Not so long ago the importance of honest and open communication when dealing with an incurable illness was largely unrecognized. We now regard it as unethical not to allow patients the opportunity to know the facts of their illness, to participate fully in decisions regarding treatment, to choose when and how to involve their families, to be given support to cope with loss, and to make choices about their terminal care. To do this well requires awareness, skill, and training. We do well to remember that doctors do not have all the answers to life, and sometimes can only listen and care. One of the most devastating statements for a patient is, 'There is nothing more we can do':

> Slowly, I learn about the importance of powerlessness.
> I experience it in my own life and I live with it in my work.
> The secret is not to be afraid of it—not to run away.
> The dying know we are not God.
> All that they ask is that we do not desert them.
>
> (S. Cassidy 1988)

CASE STUDY 2

John is a 25-year-old man with recently diagnosed end-stage lung cancer. He has difficulty controlling bone pain caused by bone secondaries. His disease is not responding to chemotherapy. He has an 18-year-old girlfriend and a 2-year-old daughter. He demands to see a doctor and wants to know why the treatment is not working and why he is still in pain. He is clearly angry. As you begin to talk he blurts out, 'I am going to die', and begins to cry. You have a frank discussion about his very limited prognosis. He decides not to go to hospital for further management of his pain despite the knowledge that there are options available. He goes home that afternoon, and spends the next few weeks with his family, and plans his wedding and the financial future of his girlfriend and daughter. He dies at home with his family and district nurse present.

Principles of breaking bad news

- Listen
- Set the scene
- Find out what the patient understands
- Find out how much information the patient wants to know
- Share information using common language
- Review and summarize
- Allow opportunity for questions
- Agree follow-up and support

Reactions to bad news

- Shock
- Anger
- Denial
- Bargaining

- Relief
- Sadness
- Fear
- Guilt
- Anxiety
- Distress

Not every patient and family will reach a stage of acceptance; indeed, for some it is important to avoid a sense of giving in:

> Do not go gently into that good night
> Old age should burn and rave at close of day
> Rage, rage against the dying of the light.
>
> *(Dylan Thomas)*

Bereavement

> No one ever told me that grief felt so like fear.
> I am not afraid, but the sensation is like being afraid.
> The same fluttering in the stomach, the same restlessness.
>
> *(C. S. Lewis)*

Grief, the emotions felt in response to bereavement, is an individual experience but there is much about the process that traces a common road. This path has been described in terms of phases or tasks (see Figure 18.2). The normal grief process may take months or years. Those facing bereavement may need support long after the funeral is over and the reassurance that they are 'normal' (see case study 3). Abnormal or distorted grief reactions can occur, if this process is suppressed either deliberately or subconsciously, and may need more expert help. Bereavement is associated with morbidity and mortality. The popular notion that 'he died of a broken heart' may have some validity. Studies are variable, but there is a consistent increase in deaths from ischaemic heart disease in widowers.

Services in the community

Hospice/home/hospital

Most people choose to die at home. However, the majority of deaths occur in the acute hospital setting. Specialist palliative care units or hospices account for 15–20% depending on the area. This high level of institutional deaths may be unavoidable with unexpected and traumatic death. When the death is

Phase	Features	Task
Denial	Shock, disbelief, sense of unreality	To accept the reality of the loss
Pain/distress	Hurt, anger, guilt, worthlessness, searching	To experience the pain of grief
Realisation	Depression, apathy, fantasy	To adjust to life without the deceased
Acceptance	Readiness to engage in new activities and relationships	To relocate emotional energy elsewhere

Fig. 18.2 Phases and tasks of grief.

CASE STUDY 3

Pat's husband died a few months ago. He had prostate cancer and then a stroke, and she had cared for him at home. They had been married for 35 years and had no children. She had coped with the funeral arrangements and sorting her husband's belongings, but now felt very alone. She was not sleeping very well, and woke to see her husband standing beside her and comforting her. These visions were very real and continued for a few weeks. She was glad to have seen him, but now came to her GP wondering if she was going mad. You spend time talking, and encouraging her to express her grief and fears. You reassure her that such hallucinations can be a normal part of the grieving process. You encourage her to contact a bereavement support group and arrange to see her again. Over the next few months Pat begins to come to terms with the loss of her husband. She finds the support of others who have had a similar experience very valuable.

---

anticipated families may feel unable to cope despite a patient's request to be at home. However, one of the major barriers to terminal care at home is poor communication between secondary and primary care. Better awareness of the services available, a multidisciplinary approach, and the use of short admissions for symptom control, respite, and shared care may help support the primary care team, as well as the patient and family. Better funding of these services is badly needed.

Euthanasia

Euthanasia means literally 'gentle' or easy death. However, the term has now come to mean the deliberate ending of a persons life with or without their request. The associated issues around the withdrawal of treatment should not be confused and the term passive euthanasia is discouraged.

Definitions

Voluntary euthanasia: deliberate ending of a person's life at their request.
Non-voluntary euthanasia: deliberate ending of a person's life without a specific request.
Physician assisted suicide: physician provides the means and advice for suicide.
In the UK euthanasia is illegal, though difficult ethical dilemmas regarding treatment decisions may need to be tested in the courts. The House of Lords Select Committee report in 1994 recommended no change in the law to permit euthanasia, and recommended the development and growth of palliative care. The issue continues to be debated at a philosophical, ethical, and legal level, and also on an individual level. In the Netherlands, the law has changed in the late 1990s to allow euthanasia under certain circumstances.

Why do patients request euthanasia?

This question is less researched than the ethical arguments for and against euthanasia. Perhaps 3–8% of patients with advanced disease will ask to die. The most common reasons are unrelieved symptoms or the dread of further suffering. Loss of control and dependency are more often cited as reasons than pain. Some studies indicate that 60% of patients requesting euthanasia may be depressed.

Response to a request for euthanasia

+ Listen
+ Acknowledge the issue
+ Explore the reasons behind the request
+ Explore ways of giving more control to the patient
+ Look for treatable problems
+ Remember spiritual issues
+ Admit powerlessness

CASE STUDY 4

Robbie is a 62-year-old ex-seaman with metastatic carcinoma of prostate. He had a number of other medical problems including peripheral vascular disease, cerebrovascular disease, and previous alcohol excess. He lives alone with little family support and separated from his usual social support, as he was too unwell to visit his local pub. He has unrelenting pain from his bone secondaries. He attempts suicide on two separate occasions, taking an overdose of opiates, antidepressants, and alcohol. After both of these attempts he was resuscitated.

CASE STUDY 4 Continued

He wants to die and asks you for euthanasia. You listen to his request and acknowledge his sense of hopelessness and failure. You explain that you cannot offer euthanasia, but may be able to help. Over the next few months Robbie's pain is much better controlled, his depression responds to treatment, and he agrees to attend the local palliative care day unit for support. He meets several of his seafaring and drinking friends again. He takes an interest again in his local football team, despite it being bottom of the league, and arranges for cable TV to be installed in his home. Robbie's disease gradually progresses and he dies in the palliative care unit at his request. He lived 18 months after his suicide attempts and did not request euthanasia again.

You matter because you are you. You matter to the last moment of your life and we will do all we can not only to help you die peacefully, but to live until you die. (Cicely Saunders)

SUMMARY POINTS

- Death is part of life, but our society tends to hide it away, although that was not the case in the past.
- The early Hippocratic tradition was not to 'challenge the gods' by attempting to treat those deemed to be incurable, but twenty-first century medicine sees death as its enemy, leading to the fear that life must be prolonged at all costs, regardless of its quality.
- Patterns of mortality have changed. In the nineteenth century more than 1 in 10 babies died and infectious diseases generally accounted for a third of all deaths. In developed countries, cancer is now a leading cause of death, mainly because more people survive long enough to experience it. Nonetheless, since the nineteenth century, life expectancy in the UK has increased by over 30 years.
- Unexpected deaths and multiple deaths (e.g. from disasters) need separate consideration because of the special reactions that they arouse, including difficulties in health professionals themselves.
- Terminal care is properly applied when the patient is faced with dying. Palliative care is applied when the patient is living through an illness. The term 'terminal illness' is misleading.
- Palliative care emphasizes quality of life, with a focus on symptom control and a holistic, team-based, and community-orientated approach.

SUMMARY POINTS Continued

- ◆ 'Euthanasia' means literally 'gentle' or 'easy' death, although it has come to mean the deliberate ending of life. It is illegal in most countries, but is currently the subject of much debate.

References and further reading

Diamond, J. (1998). *C: Because Cowards Get Cancer Too . . .* Vermilion, London.

Doyle D., Hanks, G.W.C., MacDonald, N. (1998). *Oxford Textbook of Palliative Medicine, 2nd edn.* Oxford University Press, Oxford.

Index